The PCOS Diet Plan

THE
PCOS
Diet Plan

A Natural Approach to Health for
Women with Polycystic Ovary Syndrome

Hillary Wright, M.Ed, RD

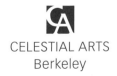

CELESTIAL ARTS
Berkeley

Library of Congress Cataloging-in-Publication Data

Wright, Hillary.
  The PCOS diet plan : a natural approach to health for women with
polycystic ovary syndrome / Hillary Wright. — 1st ed.
     p. cm.
  Summary: "A nutrition-based PCOS book that uses diet and exercise to
manage the female hormonal disorder"—Provided by publisher.
  Includes bibliographical references and index.
  1. Polycystic ovary syndrome—Popular works. 2. Polycystic ovary
syndrome—Treatment—Popular works. 3. Polycystic ovary syndrome—
Diet therapy—Popular works. I. Title. II. Title: Polycystic ovary syndrome
diet plan.
  RG480.S7W75 2010
  618.1'1—dc22
                              2010031320

ISBN 978-1-58761-023-3

Printed in the United States of America

Design by Katy Brown

10 9 8 7

First Edition

Contents

Foreword

I distinctly remember the date when Hillary Wright had her first day as the director of nutrition at the Domar Center for Mind/Body Health—it was May 1, 2006. The only reason I remember it so well is because May 1 is my birthday, and a momentous thing happened that day. We were having a staff meeting, partially to welcome Hillary, and someone had brought in a lovely chocolate cake to surprise me. I cut slices of cake for everyone, they were distributed, and then the room went still. Not a fork was lifted, and all eyes were locked on Hillary. There was no way anyone was going to eat a crumb of cake until we saw what our new nutritionist was going to do. And what did she do? She picked up her fork and took a healthy bite. With a sigh of relief, the rest of us followed suit. I am sure we all had the same thought: "Thank heavens she is not a fanatic about every calorie and seems to have a wonderful attitude toward food!"

Hillary's attitude that day is reflected in every page of her excellent new book. Her commonsense but scientifically-backed approach to helping her readers become healthier women who happen to have PCOS, rather than at-risk scared patients, comes through on every page. There are literally millions of women in this country who have no idea how to eat and live, in fact thrive, while living with PCOS, and this book will lead them through the steps carefully, accurately, and compassionately.

Many people have the expectation that there is a pill that will treat—if not cure—all diseases. Sadly, not only is this not the case with many chronic illnesses, it is also not the case for PCOS. Modern medicine has yet to discover that magic bullet. However, research does show that women who learn to eat in a different way, exercise sensibly, and keep their stress levels at a manageable level can in fact control and in some cases eliminate their symptoms. This successful holistic approach makes sense for many reasons—there are no risks or side effects, and in addition to helping you become healthier, it also helps you feel more in control of a condition which can be bewildering and confusing.

I also remember the very first patient of mine who received a diagnosis of PCOS. It was many years ago and when she first told me about her diagnosis, I was embarrassed because I didn't know much about the syndrome. I had heard the term in graduate school, and vaguely knew the symptoms. But to be honest, I felt helpless to do much to support her. So there she sat, in my office, looking at me and clearly expecting a wealth of information. I felt like I was failing her since my role in our relationship was to provide stress relief and coping skills, yet I had no idea what she had to deal with and even less of an ability to teach her how to live a healthier life. Until now, there was no resource which encompassed it all—information on the physiology of PCOS, risk factors, nutritional explanations, and incredibly straightforward and easy-to-follow meal and lifestyle plans.

Fast-forward about twenty years, and I now have the tools I need to educate my patients with PCOS because I have read this book cover to cover. Too late for my patient of years ago, but definitely not too late for you.

—Alice Domar, PhD, executive director of the Domar
Center for Mind/Body Health and director of Mind/Body
Services at Boston IVF

Acknowledgments

Without the support and encouragement of so many people, this book never would have come to be. I'd like to thank my agent, Judith Riven, who saw us through some tricky and unanticipated situations, and my editor, Sara Golski, and the staff at Ten Speed Press who showed so much respect for my work and what I was trying to produce. Thank you to my cousins Rachel Prindle and Maura Sheehan, whose guidance was invaluable and so appreciated; the very talented David Parmentier and Monica DeSalvo for bringing their artistic eyes to my manuscript; Dr. Alice Domar, Dr. Alison Zimon, and all my colleagues at the Domar Center for Mind/Body Health and Boston IVF who have helped me realize my dream, and Dr. Natalie Schultz, Larry Lindner, and Dr. Margo Woods for professional advice and encouragement in the early days of this project.

My PCOS patients have provided the ultimate inspiration for writing this book—thanks for teaching me so much; thanks also to my "Arlington girls" and my Dana Farber "team" for your wonderful friendship and support when I felt overwhelmed by life at times; thank you to my pal and professional guiding light, Elizabeth Ward, MS, RD, who's always showed by example (and with humor!) what's possible in the nutrition world.

I'd also like to thank my parents, Alan and Marie, who have always been my biggest fans; my in-laws, Jack and Nancy Holowitz; my sister, Alison, and my brothers, John, Chris, Brian, and Michael, and their families; and my amazingly supportive husband, Tony, and my beautiful boys—John, Matt, and Brian—thanks for helping me make room in my life for this. I love you.

Introduction

The first time a woman with polycystic ovary syndrome (PCOS) showed up in my office, I had no idea what to do for her. In addition to enduring many troubling symptoms of the condition, she was also struggling with infertility. It was early 2000 and I had just returned to work from maternity leave after having my third son. I'd had no problems conceiving my first child, but it had taken almost a year and a half to get pregnant with my second son after treatment for secondary infertility three years earlier. As a fertility patient myself, I understood what she was going through. I'd been through all the tests—hormone tests, an endometrial biopsy, a hysterosalpingogram (a procedure that involves blasting dye through the fallopian tubes to make sure they're open, which in some cases actually paves the way for conception even if no blockages are found), and serial HCG (pregnancy hormone) tests once I got a positive pregnancy test. The barrage of tests left my arms looking like those of an IV drug addict. Fortunately, the solution to my secondary infertility had been some relatively simple hormonal tweaking, and, interestingly, I hadn't required any intervention for my third child. But I was well aware how complicated the quest to have a child could get. This woman's course was likely to be much more complicated than mine: she was overweight, her hormones were out of whack, and her stress level was through the roof. Her treatment would involve more than a few well-timed hormone shots.

Given my personal experience with fertility challenges, I was thrilled that Dr. Natalie Schultz was interested in developing a partnership between the fertility and nutrition departments at the large medical practice in Boston where I worked as a nutritionist and she as a fertility specialist. I'd received my medical care from Natalie, and we had become close during my treatment. Besides being a fantastic physician, she was a big fan of the nutritionists in the practice, so when she also started to see women with PCOS, she looked to us for help. As nutritionists we were definitely flattered, but at the time we weren't confident that we knew how to help these women.

Back then, I had no idea what this strange-sounding condition was, never mind how diet and lifestyle could potentially affect it. But Natalie was confident that we'd make a great team and could ultimately make a difference in these women's lives. She patiently explained PCOS to me and answered my questions, as I tried to piece together some sort of diet therapy. I had my own team of nutritionists for collaboration. First was my biochemistry-whiz nutritionist colleague, Ann Stawaris, who loves nothing more than debating the virtues of enzymes and chemical pathways. Next I found New York dietitian Martha McKittrick, who willingly shared what she knew about the condition with me. I also consulted what I consider the bible on PCOS, Samuel Thatcher's *PCOS: The Hidden Epidemic*.[1]

The key to figuring out how to manage PCOS nutritionally was learning that in most cases the driving force behind the condition is insulin resistance, something I knew a lot about. Growing up, two of my five siblings had type 1 diabetes, which is caused by a lack of the pancreatic hormone insulin. Insulin resistance, a condition characterized by inefficient use of this hormone, is the cause of the more common form of diabetes in the United States, known as type 2 diabetes. This early exposure to the world of diabetes care got me interested in becoming a dietitian in the first place.

Using my knowledge of how to manage insulin resistance, I began to treat women with PCOS. Initially there were just a few patients, but over time the number has grown to several hundred. One thing became clear: the women with PCOS had many symptoms and complaints in common, and most of them felt fairly underserved by the medical profession. I realized that many nutritionists knew little about this condition, and a number of them began to look to me for guidance. I developed a presentation on managing PCOS for dietitians in my area; time and again, I would receive the same feedback: "I really know nothing about this" and "Oh my God, I think I have it!" This wasn't surprising, given that more than 97 percent of registered dietitians are female!

As we began to see more women with PCOS in our medical practice, the nutritionists and the fertility and endocrinology department began running group support classes for women with PCOS, many of whom were thrilled to have a place to finally talk about their health. A common thread for many of these women was knowing for *years* that something was wrong but never being able to get much satisfaction—or symptom relief—from their physicians. PCOS is a hormonal problem, and women would accordingly describe a wide range of physical and emotional symptoms. Many intuitively felt that their symptoms were connected, but unfortunately they frequently reported being brushed off by their doctors. Instead, they were told for the umpteenth time to lose weight and were given the impression that perhaps the problems were all in their head.

In the medical establishment's defense, at the time there just was not as much awareness of the prevalence of polycystic ovary syndrome. For these women to finally land in the hands of a health-care team that got it was an amazingly affirming experience. As positive as this sense of validation can be, however, it is unnerving to learn about the reality of what a diagnosis of PCOS can mean to a woman's overall health and fertility. Many women felt overwhelmed by the diet and lifestyle changes necessary to reduce the risks of a number of scary health problems, including diabetes and heart disease. In my experience, many women were first diagnosed with PCOS after seeking medical advice to find out why they weren't getting pregnant. It's easy to understand why they'd feel overwhelmed and stressed.

The PCOS support group we established was incredibly diverse: we had young women, older women (who were just figuring out the diagnosis despite years of fertility treatments!), straight women, gay women, teenage girls and their moms, women trying to get pregnant, and women with no interest in kids but a strong interest in avoiding diabetes. Although this diversity did make for some challenging dynamics, we kept the group going for a couple of years until the clinicians left the practice (Natalie moved to the Midwest) and the demands of our own jobs as nutritionists led to the support group's demise.

I continued to see a steady stream of PCOS patients until I left the practice in 2006 to take a part-time job at Boston's Dana Farber Cancer Institute. At this point I also established a private nutrition counseling practice that would ultimately be absorbed by the Domar Center for Mind/Body Health at Boston IVF, one of the nation's oldest and most successful fertility treatment practices in the country. I was recruited by Dr. Alice Domar, an international expert on the application of mind-body medicine to women's health issues, specifically for my expertise in the nutrition management of PCOS. I've been blessed to work alongside some amazing therapists, acupuncturists, clinicians, and support staff—all of whom are vested in the Domar Center's philosophy of providing comprehensive care that is "grounded in science, inspired by compassion."

That motto nicely frames my intentions for this book, *The PCOS Diet Plan*: to provide diet and lifestyle information that is backed by science and designed to empower women diagnosed with this condition. When applied soundly to one's own life, this information can initiate broad health and life-enhancing effects. As intimidating as it can be, PCOS is a condition that can absolutely be influenced in a positive way by diet and lifestyle. The strategies described in this book are not overrestrictive or off the wall, and they can easily be followed by anyone interested in healthy living. They require a little education on how female bodies work—or, more specifically, how women's bodies were *designed* to work—and how we can adjust diet and lifestyle to work *with* our genetic makeup in an environment that often colludes against it.

One important point to keep in mind throughout this book: learning to take better care of your health is not about "dieting." It's about modifying your behavior to incorporate lifelong healthy habits, while occasionally enjoying things that diets often tell us are forbidden. If you follow the recommendations in this book, I guarantee you'll feel better and more energetic, you'll lower your risk of diabetes and heart disease, and you'll feel more in control of your health. All this without feeling like food is the enemy but, rather, one of life's great pleasures.

PART 1

Defining Polycystic Ovary Syndrome

1

The Mystery of PCOS

Many people are unfamiliar with the strange-sounding condition of polycystic ovary syndrome (PCOS). From infertility to heart disease, the broad reach of PCOS can intimidate and overwhelm even the most health-conscious women who are up to speed on the connection between their diet, lifestyle, and health. There's a lot to learn, and a lot we still don't understand about the syndrome. Common reactions to a diagnosis of PCOS include the following:

- *Confusion.* What exactly is this condition that has the potential to affect so many aspects of my health, but that many health-care providers seem to know so little about?
- *Frustration.* Why, after complaining about my symptoms to health-care providers for years, am I just now finding out what this is? (For those trying to get pregnant, the timing couldn't be worse.) Now I have to figure out how to manage this complex condition in the hope a new diet and lifestyle will help me get pregnant.
- *Stress.* All the information is confusing, and none of it sounds good. Feeling like I have to change so many things about my lifestyle to get better is overwhelming and even paralyzing.
- *Relief.* Even though I'm not happy about having PCOS, now at least I know what I'm dealing with.
- *Motivation.* PCOS could have lasting effects on my health and fertility. I want to get a grip on my symptoms and participate fully in my care.

Although certainly no one *hopes* for a diagnosis of PCOS, if you've finally received the diagnosis, rest assured that this is a condition you can do something about. The diet and lifestyle changes that can help you manage your PCOS are not extreme recommendations. If more Americans in general (both men and women, old and young) adopted these recommendations, we'd see a decline in nearly every chronic health problem: heart disease, diabetes, obesity, high blood pressure, cancer, and possibly many others. Eating well and leading an active lifestyle have such far-reaching effects on one's health and quality of life: more energy, improved mood, better sleep, improved self- and body image, better sex, and less stress, to name just a few benefits.

A certain amount of the stress many people feel comes from the knowledge that they're not doing all they can to protect their health. Starting to chip away at the list of things we know we should be doing offers a certain amount of relief in itself. The diet and lifestyle recommendations outlined throughout this book are solid, healthful ideas that anyone can follow. With a diagnosis of PCOS, you just have more of an incentive to make these changes.

The Facts about PCOS

PCOS is the most common female hormonal disorder and the primary cause of anovulatory infertility (infertility caused by lack of regular ovulation). The syndrome has been recognized as having damaging lifelong health effects. PCOS is estimated to affect 5 to 10 percent of all women during their reproductive years. According to the 2000 U.S. Census, there are more than 140 million females in the United States—that's up to 14 million women who may develop the condition during their lifetime. Research suggests that up to 30 percent of women experience some symptoms of the disorder, referred to as nonclassic or variant PCOS. With the dramatic increase in childhood obesity, which often leads to earlier onset menstruation, PCOS is starting to show up in younger girls. That means more years to live with the damaging health consequences of this syndrome that never goes away. It is a lifelong, chronic condition.

The cause of PCOS is not clearly understood, but it's believed to be a complex genetic disorder likely involving multiple genes. The genes involved may be those that regulate function of the hypothalamus, the pituitary gland, and the ovaries, as well as those genes responsible for insulin resistance, which is believed to be the driving force for most of the signs and symptoms of the disorder. In fact, women with PCOS experience similar risk for the development of metabolic and cardiovascular problems as those diagnosed with metabolic syndrome, another common and complex health problem that is escalating in the U.S. population and driving the national epidemic of diabetes and heart disease. This makes sense: insulin resistance is a contributing factor in both conditions.[1]

Depending on the research you read, anywhere from 50 to 80 percent of women with PCOS are overweight or obese. The incidence of PCOS in the U.S. population has paralleled the increase in obesity, suggesting a strong connection between body weight and the severity of the condition. Although obesity has not been identified as a cause of PCOS, carrying around excess weight worsens its signs and symptoms. Women with the syndrome often store fat around the middle, known as visceral adiposity, which basically means that they tend to wrap excess body fat around their internal organs. This type of body fat storage is genetic, known to aggravate insulin resistance, and raise blood pressure and the risk of heart disease.

PCOS can also trigger a host of physical symptoms, most of which are caused by excessive production of androgens, or male-type hormones, like testosterone. The hallmark of insulin resistance is higher circulating levels of insulin, which can have a seriously toxic effect on hormone production in the ovaries. Higher circulating insulin levels increase the release of an important reproductive hormone called luteinizing hormone (LH) from the pituitary gland. Both LH and insulin then stimulate the theca cells in the ovaries to produce testosterone, which is toxic to egg development. Production of testosterone doesn't make you any less of a woman. All women make some testosterone (and all men produce some estrogen), but in the ovaries estrogen should predominate over testosterone. When excess insulin stimulates a cascade effect where testosterone predominates over estrogen, eggs don't develop normally.[2] Physical signs that androgen levels may be atypical include excess hair growth on the face, chest, and back (male-pattern growth); thinning of the hair on the crown of the head; acne; and a tendency to gain much-maligned "belly fat" (an apple-shaped body as opposed to the healthier pear-shaped body, where body fat is stored more in the buttocks and thighs).

Women with PCOS are also at greater risk of a number of life-threatening chronic health problems. Most concerning is the connection between PCOS and type 2 diabetes. Diabetes is exploding in the U.S. population. Type 2 diabetes has increased 40 percent since the early 2000s. Undiagnosed diabetes is seven times more likely in women with PCOS, compared with similar-age women without the condition. In fact, 30 to 40 percent of women with PCOS have prediabetes (that is, they don't yet have full-blown diabetes, but they are already showing signs of insulin resistance, which causes type 2 diabetes). As many as 10 percent of women with PCOS develop full-blown diabetes by age forty.[3] A recently released report published in the journal *Diabetes Care* suggests that over the next twenty-five years, the number of Americans living with diabetes will nearly double, increasing from 23.7 million in 2009 to 44.1 million in 2034. Over the same period, spending on diabetes will almost triple, rising from $113 billion to $336 billion, even with no increase in the prevalence of obesity.[4]

Heart disease continues to be the number-one killer of both women and men in the United States, and women with PCOS have a four to seven times higher risk of heart attack than women of the same age without the syndrome.[5] Endometrial cancer is also a risk for women with PCOS. The hormone estrogen triggers the growth of cells that line the uterus, which are usually shed once a month due to the opposing effect of the hormone progesterone. But in cases of PCOS, where periods are inconsistent or absent, the lining of the uterus builds up, raising the risk of endometrial hyperplasia (overgrowth of the endometrium), which down the road may lead to endometrial cancer. Hyperinsulinemia (elevated blood levels of insulin due to insulin resistance) is common in PCOS and can encourage the growth of potentially cancerous cells. If left untreated, research suggests that endometrial hyperplasia advances to endometrial cancer in as many as 30 percent of cases.[6]

With many women having children later in life, the number of women requiring fertility treatment is also on the rise, and the hormonal changes seen in PCOS have been recognized to be a major player in the world of infertility. If a woman with PCOS does become pregnant, she's at higher risk of gestational (pregnancy-induced) diabetes, which presents a risk to both the mother and the developing baby. Some research suggests that women with PCOS are three times more likely to miscarry than women without the disorder.

Another threatening aspect of PCOS is that although 5 to 30 percent of women may have PCOS or some of its symptoms, awareness about the syndrome—even among many health-care providers—remains inadequate. The emergence of information on the prevalence of the syndrome is very much like what happened with fibromyalgia and hypothyroidism in the 1990s. Prior to these disorders being recognized as affecting large numbers of women, many women—and clinicians—failed to recognize the symptoms as a collection of complaints caused by one underlying health problem. Today, both disorders are widely recognized as treatable, as is PCOS.

A Historical Look at PCOS

In the medical literature the earliest mention of polycystic ovary syndrome dates back more than 150 years to France, where the first official description of polycystic-appearing ovaries was made in 1845. In the early 1900s a few isolated reports began to emerge describing a procedure called a wedge resection (the removal of a section of the ovary) used to treat cystic changes in the ovaries, but knowledge was still very much isolated to treating the ovarian cysts. An understanding of the systemic reach of the condition was still years away.[7] In 1935 the American gynecologists Irving Stein and Michael Leventhal published a paper on their findings in seven women with amenorrhea (the absence of menstruation), hirsutism (excessive thick hair growth in male-pattern areas), obesity, and cystic-appearing ovaries. This was one of the first descriptions of the complex condition known today as PCOS, which at the time was termed Stein-Leventhal syndrome after the trailblazing physicians who had first tied the symptoms together.[8] Because of the ovary's cystic appearance, Stein and Leventhal referred to the condition as polycystic ovarian *disease*, but as more was learned about PCOS, the term "syndrome" began to emerge.

Although it is appropriately named a syndrome, the fact that PCOS is a syndrome as opposed to a disease contributes to much of the confusion around diagnosing it. What is the difference between a syndrome and a disease? Let's start by looking at technical definitions of the two terms: a *disease* is a pathological condition of a part, organ, or system of an organism resulting from various causes and characterized by an identifiable group of signs or symptoms; a *syndrome* is a group of symptoms that collectively indicates or characterizes a disease or another abnormal condition, the cause of which may or may not be known, and for which no single test is diagnostic.

While these definitions basically sound the same, the difference is in the details. A disease has an "identifiable group of signs or symptoms" that you either have or you don't. To be diagnosed with a disease, you have to meet all the criteria. A syndrome is different in that there could be a number of signs and symptoms that vary between individuals, and potentially indicate a condition, but not all signs and symptoms have to be met to make a diagnosis. In other words, there may be a list of potential signs and symptoms, and if you have enough of them, your clinician may say you have the condition. (A similar condition is IBS, irritable bowel syndrome, where physicians generally rule out more serious gastrointestinal diseases and end up with a diagnosis of IBS.) It is critical to be evaluated by a physician who's used to seeing patients with PCOS—his or her clinical judgment and experience seeing hundreds of women presenting with a similar constellation of symptoms may allow the physician to pull together a clinical picture that might not be as apparent to someone with less experience diagnosing the condition. That doesn't mean all those doctors who missed the diagnosis were bad doctors; they likely weren't used to seeing a lot of women with PCOS. In their defense, it's only been since the early 2000s or so that the prevalence and importance of treating this syndrome has come to light.

Symptoms of PCOS and Getting a Diagnosis

A woman may see her doctor for several reasons that may ultimately result in a diagnosis of PCOS. Her menstrual periods may not come on a regular basis—or at all—a condition called amenorrhea. Or she's been trying to get pregnant without success. She may be experiencing unwanted hair growth, severe acne, or weight problems—all of which are negatively affecting her body image and self-esteem. She may have been diagnosed with some metabolic abnormality, such as elevated blood sugar (glucose), high cholesterol, or high blood pressure, often at a young age. She may just have a feeling that "something isn't right" with her body, and she's hoping a doctor can pull it together for her.

Scientists don't know exactly what causes PCOS. No single factor can account for the array of abnormalities seen in the syndrome, but research suggests that the underlying primary cause in most cases is insulin resistance—a condition that responds strongly to weight loss, exercise, a healthful diet, and medications when necessary. We do know that PCOS is a genetic condition, likely complicated by ovarian and metabolic abnormalities that, when taken together, can create a potential firestorm of health risks. This is particularly true when environmental factors like obesity, an unhealthy diet, and a sedentary lifestyle are stirred into the mix. Further complicating matters, it appears there are different phenotypes or genetically different forms of PCOS.[9] Some phenotypes are at higher risk of diabetes and other metabolic problems (those with apple-body obesity and signs of insulin resistance), and others appear at lower risk (thin women with PCOS and no evidence of androgen excess). Women with classic PCOS—those with spotty or absent periods and androgen excess—are more likely to have more severe insulin resistance and other metabolic problems.

There are differing opinions on the criteria for a diagnosis of PCOS. Regardless of criteria used, the first step is to rule out related disorders, such as Cushing's Syndrome and Congenital Adrenal Hyperplasia (CAH). The main criteria used to diagnose the syndrome tends to run along continental lines, with physicians in the United States preferring criteria set during the 1990 National Institutes of Health (NIH) International Conference on PCOS. European physicians tend to favor the more recent 2003 consensus developed by the European Society for Human Reproduction and Embryology and the American Society for Reproductive Medicine, called the Rotterdam Criteria, named after the city in which the criteria were drafted. In 2006 an international organization called the Androgen Excess and PCOS Society weighed in with their own criteria that attempted to meld together the NIH and Rotterdam Criteria, basically concluding that hyperandrogenism is the cornerstone of PCOS but also conceding the possibility that there are forms of PCOS without blatant evidence of hyperandrogenism that need more study.[10]

1990 NIH Criteria for PCOS

To be diagnosed with PCOS you must meet *all* the following criteria:		
Hyperandrogenism	Oligo-ovulation	Exclusion of related disorders

2003 Rotterdam Criteria for PCOS

To be diagnosed with PCOS you must have two of the following criteria:		
Oligo-ovulation or anovulation	Clinical or biochemical signs of hyperandrogenism	Polycystic ovaries

For the 1990 criteria the NIH held an international conference on PCOS and basically took a show of hands on what the audience and speakers thought should be included in the criteria. The consensus was, to be diagnosed with PCOS, after other disorders were ruled out, a woman had to have these two complaints: (1) chronic oligoanovulation (few or no periods) and (2) biochemical or clinical signs of excess androgen (excess hair growth, thinning of the hair on the head, and so on). Interestingly, having polycystic ovaries visible on ultrasound was not required to be present for diagnosis, which was basically a nod to the belief that ovaries were only *part* of the picture, despite the syndrome's name.

In an effort to be more inclusive—and to recognize that the diagnosis may be broader than these two criteria— the Rotterdam Criteria expanded the diagnosis of PCOS to women if they met two of the following three conditions: (1) oligoanovulation or anovulation, (2) the clinical or biochemical diagnosis of androgen excess, and (3) polycystic ovaries visible on ultrasound. Because the Rotterdam Criteria uses the presence of cystic ovaries as one of the criteria that can be present to diagnose PCOS, it opens the diagnosis pool up to women with normal periods and fertility but who have signs of androgen excess and polycystic ovaries on ultrasound as well as to women who have irregular periods and polycystic ovaries but no signs of androgen excess. This expanded criterion is believed to increase the number of women who could be diagnosed with PCOS by about 20 percent. Although this categorization sounds confusing, it may clarify the confusion for women who might doubt their PCOS diagnosis because they're thin (many of the books and online information women read about PCOS suggest they're more likely to be overweight if they have PCOS) and without signs of androgen excess but have irregular periods and cystic ovaries on ultrasound.

In addition to adding phenotypes beyond "classic PCOS," the Rotterdam Criteria includes many more women who have milder PCOS symptoms and are less likely to be overweight, many of whom are probably less affected by the metabolic abnormalities (insulin resistance, high cholesterol, and so on) seen in classic PCOS. The 2006 Androgen Excess and PCOS Society criteria are worth mentioning, although they don't change the picture much. Their position accepts the NIH criteria with some modifications based on the concerns of the Rotterdam Criteria, basically concluding that hyperandrogenism is the cornerstone of PCOS but also conceding the possibility there are forms of PCOS without blatant evidence of hyperandrogenism that need more study. Acknowledging the criteria will evolve over time as new findings emerge, they officially concluded that until more is known, all three of the following criteria should be present to diagnose PCOS: (1) hyperandrogenism (excess hair growth and/or blood tests suggesting high androgens); (2) ovarian dysfunction (lack of regular periods and/or polycystic ovaries); and (3) exclusion of other androgen excess or related disorders.

Particularly if you're looking for a reason *not* to have PCOS, it can be overwhelming and confusing. But identifying all these different "types" of PCOS begs the question, do we treat women who have a diagnosis of PCOS but who don't have all the classic signs and symptoms the same? And what about the fact that gaining or losing weight could move a woman in and out of criteria because of its effect on ovulation and androgen production? Until we know more about the degree to which these less-classic cases of the syndrome may be affected by insulin resistance—the primary abnormality affecting women with PCOS—the prudent thing to do is to assume some increased risk and fine-tune diet and lifestyle accordingly. If we look at irregular periods, excess androgens, and polycystic ovaries as three variables to be mixed and matched, it's possible there may be differences in how women should be treated based on their life and health goals. Scientists say some degree of insulin resistance can be assumed once someone's Body Mass Index (BMI) drifts over 30 (the clinical definition of obesity). According to a 2005–2006 survey from the Centers for Disease Control and Prevention (CDC), 35.3 percent of women in the United States are obese—all of whom would benefit from the information presented in this book (even without a diagnosis of PCOS).

The Clinician and PCOS Diagnosis

It's important to be fully evaluated by a health-care provider who has considerable PCOS experience. This may be your primary care provider—be it a medical doctor, a physician's assistant, or a nurse practitioner—or an endocrinology specialist. According to PCOS expert Dr. Samuel Thatcher, in no other gynecological condition is a thorough medical history more important than in PCOS. Knowing what questions to ask—and a willingness to listen as you tell your story—is critical to helping piece together whether you have PCOS. No one knows your history better than you. You're looking to form a partnership, so don't settle for being brushed aside by a busy clinician looking to cut to the chase. The sidebar on page 18, written by reproductive endocrinologist Dr. Alison Zimon, includes information on obtaining a comprehensive medical evaluation for PCOS. Zimon outlines the type of information your doctor will gather from your medical history and physical exam as well as the tests you might expect and medications that might be helpful depending on your circumstances.

Using Medications to Manage PCOS

My goal is to help you manage your health and hormones as naturally as possible through diet and lifestyle change (by boosting activity, taking sensible supplements, managing stress, and so on). But despite your best efforts, sometimes medications are needed to help regulate your menstrual cycles, control your symptoms, manage your health risk factors, or just to help you see your way clear to what needs to happen to get better. Medications can be used as an ally on the road to better health. Some problems, like hypothyroidism, don't respond to diet or exercise. Or perhaps what's happening with your health has been going on for a while and has progressed to the point where you need to start medications to get better. Maybe you're showing signs of prediabetes, and medications may help reduce the risk of progressing to full-blown diabetes.

There is also the possibility of starting out on medications you may be able to wean off of down the road, as the effects of diet and lifestyle change take hold. Or you may only need medications temporarily (to increase your odds of getting pregnant, for example). But medications can never compensate for a lousy diet and sedentary lifestyle—that is, you can't take meds instead of making diet and lifestyle changes and expect to get the optimal results from the medications. Many people with diabetes have run through a long list of oral agents to manage the disease, only to eventually end up on insulin. Sometimes, try as you might, things turn out this way, but there's a lot we can do to keep our dependence on medications to a minimum.

Medications used to treat PCOS tend to fall into several categories (see the table below): insulin sensitizers, hormone regulators, symptom management meds, lipid (cholesterol)-lowering meds, and blood pressure regulators.

Medications to Treat PCOS

MEDICATION	EXAMPLE
Insulin sensitizers	metformin, pioglitazone, rosiglitazone
Hormone regulators	oral contraceptive pills, progesterone, clomiphene citrate, letrozol
Symptom management	spirinolactone, finasteride, minoxidil, retonoin, tetracycline
Lipid (cholesterol)-lowering agents	gemfibrozil, niacin, statins
Blood pressure regulators	diuretics, angiotensin-enzyme inhibitors, angiotensin-receptor blockers, beta-blockers, calcium channel blockers

Preparing for the Doctor's Visit

In today's health-care environment, many physicians are crunched for time. Be sure to bring anything to the appointment that outlines your past medical history and specific concerns. Make a list of all the potentially important pieces of the puzzle for the PCOS expert to analyze. This greatly facilitates the gathering of information and helps the clinician develop a clear picture of what's been happening and what your goals are. Gather the following information ahead of time:

- **Menstrual history.** How old were you when you got your first period? What has your menstrual pattern been like? Are there any previous pregnancies, and if so, how many?
- **Weight history.** If you are currently overweight, did your weight change significantly in a short period of time? Has your weight been a challenge all your life, or has managing it become more of a problem recently?

- **Family history.** Are there diabetes, heart disease, cancer, history of fertility problems, or weight issues in your family?
- **Medications and/or dietary supplements.** Include everything you are taking as well as the doses.
- **Previous tests.** If available, bring along the results of previous blood tests, ultrasounds, and so on.

The first thing that will generally happen in the diagnosis process is that the doctor will look to rule out other explanations for your health complaints. These might include such disorders as hyperprolactinmeia, nonclassic congenital adrenal hyperplasia, or Cushing's syndrome, a hormonal disorder caused by prolonged exposure of the body's tissues to high levels of the hormone cortisol. The doctor will weed through three different types of information: the symptoms and a physical examination, a variety of blood tests, and other test results. What exactly is he or she looking for?

Menstrual Disturbances

Women with PCOS typically get their periods around the usual age of twelve to thirteen, but it's not uncommon for a young woman to make her first trip to the gynecologist because she hasn't gotten her period at all. Menstruation may start out regular, but by the mid-teens cycles may start to lengthen or be skipped altogether. Frequently, birth control pills are prescribed to regulate this, but this doesn't mean the PCOS is gone. The symptoms are just being overridden by the hormones in the oral contraceptives. During the teen years skin problems seen in women with PCOS may also start to kick in (although acne in general isn't unusual during the teen years).

Because oral contraceptives regulate hormones, and therefore many of the signs and symptoms of PCOS, it's not unusual for a woman to think all is well—until she goes off her birth control pills for one reason or another and then she doesn't get her period. Although some women with PCOS have fairly regular twenty-eight-day cycles, PCOS should be suspected in anyone with cycles that last longer than thirty-five days. Those women without periods will often be given medications (like progestin) to trigger the onset of a period. Age at menopause is believed to be the same for women with and without PCOS.

Skin and Hair Problems

Skin problems in women with PCOS are extremely common, brought on by increased levels of male hormones (androgens). Androgens increase production of sebum (an oily substance secreted by the sebaceous glands in

What to Expect from Your Doctor

By Dr. Alison Zimon, reproductive endocrinologist at Boston IVF

A complete workup for PCOS will involve ruling out a number of conditions that can masquerade as PCOS in their presentation and will confirm the PCOS diagnosis. It will also address the severity of your PCOS and its associated health problems, including impaired glucose tolerance, diabetes, obesity, high cholesterol, infertility, hypertension, and cardiac disease. Most commonly, particularly in the United States, the diagnosis is made when a woman has less frequent or absent menstrual cycles with evidence for excess male hormones and other conditions are excluded. A comprehensive evaluation will likely include a detailed focused history of your symptoms, your health, and your family's health. Your clinician may ask about your pubertal milestones, menstrual patterns, weight fluctuations, signs of excess male hormones (such as acne and excess hair growth), and other medical conditions and symptoms. A physical exam will be performed and, in addition to a routine exam, will include screening for signs of male hormone excess, abnormal endocrine function, insulin resistance, reproductive development, and anatomic abnormalities.

Your clinician may conclude that you have PCOS based on your history and exam alone. However, often he or she will order tests to complete the evaluation or send you to a specialist for this. Most likely, these will include serum measurements of luteinizing hormone (LH) and follicle stimulating hormone (FSH), which are hormones secreted from the pituitary gland in the brain that regulate ovarian function. Levels of the ovarian hormone (estrogen) and the male hormones (testosterone, androstenedione, and dehydroepiandrosterone sulfate [DHEAS]) may be measured. Some testing to evaluate your glucose and insulin metabolism may be performed, such as fasting serum glucose and insulin, glucose-load challenge, and glycosylated hemoglobin level. Most other tests will be done if alternative diagnoses are considered or need to be ruled out, including thyroid disease, excess prolactin, Cushing's disease, enzyme defects, hormone-secreting tumors, or hyperlipidemia. Your clinician may also order tests to make sure your liver and kidneys are functioning properly. Finally, if it has been six months to a year since your last period, your clinician may want to be sure you have not developed an overgrowth of your uterine lining, resulting in endometrial hyperplasia or early endometrial cancer. He or she may recommend an ultrasound to measure the lining or perform a simple office biopsy to sample the lining tissue.

the skin), which increases inflammation and bacterial growth in the skin, causing acne. Seborrhea (flaky skin) and hidradenitis suppurtiva (inflammation of the sweat glands in the armpit and groin) are also common in PCOS, as is a particularly telling skin sign called acanthosis nigricans (AN). AN is a skin condition characterized by velvety, raised, pigmented skin changes most commonly seen on the back of the neck, armpits, groin, and beneath the breasts. AN is often described as the skin "looking dirty," but the discoloration can't be scrubbed off. Skin tags are also often present. AN is frequently a skin symptom of insulin resistance and is more common in dark-skinned people.

Another major PCOS sign that can be particularly annoying is hirsutism. All manner of expensive or uncomfortable therapies exist to deal with this hair growth (laser, electrolysis, waxing, shaving)—most women will do whatever it takes—as do some medications (that either treat the underlying hormonal problems or the hair growth itself). As if growing facial hair wasn't upsetting enough, some women also experience hair thinning on the crown of the head similar to male-pattern balding. For many women a full head of hair is vital to their self-esteem, and losing it, particularly during the reproductive years, can result in nothing short of panic! The mechanism isn't completely understood, but hormones are the likely culprit. Hair loss may improve with treatment of the underlying insulin resistance. I remember one patient who started taking metformin, a medication to manage insulin resistance, and a multivitamin at the same time; she commented that the vitamin seemed to be making her hair grow thicker. The more likely explanation, however, was that her insulin levels were improving on the metformin, causing a drop in her androgen levels. Other medications exist to help mediate hair loss for women with PCOS.

Weight Problems

Being overweight or obese is commonly associated with PCOS, but which comes first, the chicken or the egg? Likely, it's a little bit of both—depending on individual circumstances. Research cites some widely fluctuating numbers on this, but it appears that between 50 to 80 percent of women with PCOS are overweight or obese. And they tend to carry much of their excess weight as abdominal fat (the apple versus the pear body). This is particularly damaging to overall health because of its association

Helpful Medications to Treat PCOS

By Dr. Alison Zimon, reproductive endocrinologist at Boston IVF

Insulin sensitizers. Insulin resistance is believed to be a central cause of PCOS. Insulin sensitizers (medications that make you less resistant to insulin) are sometimes used as a component of the treatment plan. The most commonly prescribed insulin sensitizer for PCOS is metformin (Glucophage); others include pioglitazone (Actos) and rosiglitazone (Avandia). They work by multiple complex mechanisms, but put simply, these medications partially reverse the insulin resistance so that the same level of insulin is better able to do its job, including driving glucose into cells. Ultimately, this lowers the body's need for insulin, the circulating levels of insulin decrease, and the demands on the pancreas are lessened. Although insulin sensitizers help the body deal with excess sugar, they rely on a healthy pancreas to secrete insulin and a healthy diet to minimize the stress of an oversupply of carbohydrates.

Hormone regulators. Depending on your menstrual patterns and your reproductive plans, medications that help normalize reproductive hormones may be prescribed. Most women with PCOS have irregular cycles and experience menses at random intervals, from thirty days to fifty days to several months or even years. This irregularity is often associated with hard-to-manage heavy and dysfunctional bleeding. Furthermore, a woman who has rare to absent menses is at risk of an overgrowth of the uterine lining (the endometrium) as a result of unopposed estrogen (in the absence of the protective postovulatory hormone progesterone). If long-standing, unopposed estrogen can lead to endometrial hyperplasia, precancer, or cancer.

Although improved diet, exercise, and concomitant weight loss can promote cycle regulation in women with PCOS, often hormone therapy is required to do this. One method is oral contraceptive pills (OCPs), because they provide a balance of estrogen and progesterone while causing a regular shedding of the lining, both of which are protective. Birth control pills, in addition to contraception, have additional benefits for women with PCOS—most notably a reduction in serum male hormones, which may help decrease acne and excess sexual hair growth (hair on the face, abdomen, inner thighs, and back). Intermittent progesterone therapy is an alternative option for women with medical contraindications to OCPs, who poorly tolerate them, or who prefer not to be on a daily hormone treatment. The progesterone Medroxyprogesterone acetate (Provera) is given for ten to fourteen days every two to four months. This therapy does not provide contraception, and a pregnancy test must be done after every interval before starting a dose. It important to keep track of the treatment schedule because to protect oneself from unopposed estrogen, a menstrual bleed must occur at least four times a year.

Sometimes improved insulin sensitivity—through weight loss, exercise, and possible insulin-sensitizing agents—will promote ovulation in a woman with PCOS. However, conception rates can be dramatically increased by using medications that induce ovulation. These work by temporarily blocking estrogen, resulting in an exaggerated stimulation of the ovary via the brain hormone follicle stimulating hormone (FSH). Two classes of these medications are selective estrogen reuptake modulators (SERMS), such as clomiphene citrate (Clomid), and aromatase inhibitors, such as letrozole (Femara). Pregnancy rates with these medications are 5 to 12 percent on average, with a 5 to 10 percent chance of a twin pregnancy.

Symptom management. Because of irregular menstrual cycles and anovulation in women with PCOS, another consequence is a hormone imbalance in the ovaries and adrenal glands marked by an excess of androgens (male hormones), including testosterone, dehydroepiandrosterone (DHEA), and androstenedione. In women a relatively modest increase in androgens overstimulates the sebaceous glands and the hair follicles on the face, neck, chest, abdomen, inner thighs, and back. As a result, many women with PCOS suffer from acne and hirsutism (excess male-pattern hair). OCPs help to lower the androgen levels and serve as the first-line therapy for hyperandrogenism. If OCPs do not achieve acceptable improvement, second-line medications may be used. Severe acne may be treated with antiproliferation medications like isoretinoin (Accutane) or antimicrobials (for example, tetracycline). Medications for treatment of hirsutism act by decreasing the hair-follicle response to androgens; Spironolactone (also a diuretic) is the most common of these. Less frequently, androgen excess in PCOS women is marked by male-pattern balding. Medical therapy is limited but acts to disrupt testosterone effect at the hair follicle and includes finasteride (Propecia) or to stimulate follicle growth as with minoxidil (Rogaine).

Lipid (cholesterol)-lowering medications. Hyperlipidemias (that is, hypercholesterolemia or hypertriglyceridemia) are significantly more common in women with PCOS. Lifestyle modifications are often a successful first-line approach and include dietary changes to lower cholesterol and increase dietary fiber, weight loss if overweight, and daily exercise. If lipid-lowering goals are not met with lifestyle changes, then medical therapy may be started. High triglycerides are treated with fibtrates (for example, gemfibrozil) or niacin, both of which may be used as first-line therapy for mild hypercholesterolemia. Most commonly, such statins as simvastatin (Zocor), pravastatin (Pravachol), and atorvastatin (Lipitor) are prescribed to achieve more pronounced cholesterol lowering.

Blood pressure regulators. Women with PCOS are two to three times more likely to develop high blood pressure or hypertension. Weight loss, dietary sodium restriction, limited alcohol consumption, and exercise comprise the first-line approach. If unsuccessful, antihypertensive medications are started. The standard medical therapies for hypertension include diuretics (hydrochlorothiazide); calcium channel blockers, like nifedine (Procardia) and amlopidine (Norvasc); angiotensin-converting enzyme inhibitors, such as lisinopril (Zestril) and enalopril (Vasotec); angiotensin-receptor blockers, like losartan (Cozaar) and irbesartan (Avapro); and beta-blockers, like labetolol and metoprol. For women with PCOS who would like to become pregnant, it is preferable to start medications with proven safety in pregnancy, such as methyl-dopa or nifedipine.[11]

with a greater risk of diabetes, hypertension, and cardiovascular disease. Certainly, there are both lean and obese women with PCOS, but obese women are more likely to be harmed by the syndrome's health implications. Likely because of a slew of metabolic derangements, many women with PCOS gain weight very easily and struggle more to lose it. Understandably, they feel frustrated, particularly when a physician stares at them cynically when they've reported having "really tried" to lose weight without results!

Obesity is so common in the United States (some scientists have called ours an obesity-promoting culture) that it's difficult to separate how much of a woman's weight problem might be due to PCOS versus the contributing factors tied to weight gain in the general population. Women with PCOS are exposed to the same influences we all are, but they may be more susceptible to their harmful effects. These realities include the following:

- Too little daily physical activity.
- Too few occupations that require "heavy lifting," contributing to progressive loss of muscle mass over time.
- Food portions that are too large given many people's sedentary lifestyle.
- Too much access to calorie-dense junk food that is loaded with calories but provides little to no nutritional benefit.
- Low intakes of whole fruits, vegetables, and whole grains, which fill you up without weighing you down with calories.
- Too little attention to the importance of eating on a regular basis, resulting in reactive overeating (usually in the evening) because we're starved when we finally get around to it!
- Too much sugar and other processed carbohydrates that shoot your insulin levels up and down, resulting in subsequent increased cravings for more sugar.

This last point presents a particular problem for women with PCOS because they often overproduce insulin anyway, and eating too much sugar and refined carbohydrates is like pouring lighter fluid on a fire. It creates an ever-increasing demand for insulin in a body that's already having trouble managing it. Some of the metabolic derangements seen in PCOS can encourage the deposition of body fat and trigger mood swings and blood sugar fluctuations that can set the stage for overeating. Among its many functions, insulin resistance tends to jog your appetite, particularly for carbohydrates. Trying to control hunger without controlling insulin response is likely to be a futile exercise in willpower.

Tests for PCOS

PCOS is a risk factor for cardiovascular disease, and as such you should be regularly screened for high blood pressure (hypertension), a condition often referred as the silent killer because of its lack of symptoms. Checking blood pressure should be a part of everyone's annual physical exam. A normal blood pressure is in the 120/80 range—the 120 being the systolic (the top number of the reading) and the 80 being the diastolic (the bottom number). Many of us have "white coat syndrome," where our blood pressure bumps up in the doctor's office because of anxiety associated with the visit but is lower at home. Studies show that people with white coat syndrome are more likely to eventually develop high blood pressure. If this sounds like you, buy a reliable battery-operated home blood pressure monitor and track your readings at different times of the day. Doctors love when patients come in with a blood pressure log in hand. It can offer important insight into what's going on between appointments.

Blood Tests

There's no single blood test for PCOS. In the eye of the experienced clinician, however, findings from a variety of tests that have strong associations with the disorder can provide hints. As a general rule, blood testing should be done in the morning, early in your menstrual cycle (your clinician will tell you when to have them done). Exactly what tests to order may vary depending on individual circumstances. When discussing test results, it's important to note that exact levels of "normal" often vary a bit between labs.

Fasting glucose. In this test, blood is drawn after a ten-hour fast to screen for prediabetes or diabetes. The results are interpreted as follows: 99 milligrams per deciliter (mg/dl) or less is considered normal; 100–125 mg/dl points to prediabetes; and 126 mg/dl or more on two different days means diabetes. Another test that may be offered is the oral glucose tolerance test (OGTT). The OGTT requires fasting for at least eight hours before the test. The plasma glucose level is measured immediately before and two hours after drinking a liquid containing seventy-five grams of glucose dissolved in water. The results are interpreted as shown in the table below. Another test that may be ordered is a glycosylated hemoglobin or hemoglobin A1C, which reflects your average glucose over the previous three months.

2-HOUR PLASMA GLUCOSE RESULT (MG/DL)	DIAGNOSIS
139 and below	Normal
140 to 199	Prediabetes (impaired glucose tolerance)
200 and above	Diabetes

Fasting lipid profile. Most people refer to this as a cholesterol test. According to the National Institutes of Health's National Cholesterol Education Program, after a nine- to twelve-hour fast, the following levels are desirable: total cholesterol below 200 mg/dl; LDL (the "bad" cholesterol) should be below 130 mg/dl, with no cardiac risk factors; HDL (the "good" cholesterol) should be 60 mg/dl or above; and triglycerides (fat in the blood) should be below 150 mg/dl.[12] Your physician may also order another test to assess risk of cardiovascular disease called a C-reactive protein (CRP). This protein is considered a marker for inflammation.

Your physician may also order a host of tests to check various hormone levels.

Follicle stimulating hormone (FSH). This is a gonadotropin produced by the pituitary gland that stimulates follicles to grow. Levels start to rise as women get closer to menopause. In general, a level above ten is high. This can be an important indicator of PCOS when considered as part of the LH to FSH ratio.

Luteinizing hormone (LH). This is the other gonadotropin produced by the pituitary that triggers ovulation (it's what ovulation predictor kits measure). LH levels are generally lower than FSH.

Free testosterone. This is familiar as a male hormone but present in smaller amounts in women. It has to be "free," or unbound to sex hormone binding globulin (SHBG), to exert its effects. It may also be measured in the free and bound forms (total testosterone). Elevations are responsible for skin and hair symptoms in women with PCOS and contribute to increased cardiovascular risk.

Sex hormone binding globulin (SHBG). This binds testosterone, so low levels mean increased amounts of testosterone are available to exert their effect around the body. Low levels can indicate insulin resistance. Women with hypothyroidism can also have low SHBG levels.

DHEA (dehydroepiandrosterone) and DHEAS (dehydroepiandrosterone sulfate). These are weak androgens produced by the adrenal glands. Their presence can indicate whether PCOS may have adrenal involvement.

Androstenedione. This is an androgen produced in the ovary and the adrenal glands.

Estrogen. This is the primary female sex hormone.

Thyroid stimulating hormone (TSH). Thyroid problems are not uncommon in women with PCOS. TSH stimulates the thyroid to make T3 and T4, hormones that help control your body's metabolism. Symptoms of hypothyroidism may mimic those seen in PCOS.

Testing for Insulin Resistance

The tricky thing about diagnosing insulin resistance is that there's no simple, accurate, readily available test. Fasting insulin levels are available and are often ordered as part of standard testing for PCOS, but they are of limited use because of the lack of universal agreement on how to interpret them. There is no standardization of fasting insulin tests (as there is with glucose and cholesterol tests, for example), so values obtained from different labs aren't comparable. Some may say that anything over 20 microunits per milliliter suggests insulin resistance, whereas others may say that anything in the teens might be abnormal. Different labs and different clinicians seem to have their own cutoff points. Despite its limitations, however, a fasting insulin value is often considered as part of the big laboratory and clinical picture.

Getting an Ultrasound

Studies suggest that transvaginal ultrasound detects polycystic ovaries in about 75 percent of women with PCOS.[13] For the Rotterdam and Androgen Society PCOS diagnostic criteria, polycystic-appearing ovaries are included as potentially part of the determining data. Ultrasounds are safe and can determine the number and size of ovarian follicles. By the current definition, a woman can be diagnosed as having polycystic ovaries if at least one ovary has an ovarian volume of greater than 10 mm³, or twelve or more follicles measuring two to nine millimeters in diameter. Because many women have polycystic ovaries without meeting the criteria for PCOS, it's important that whoever is doing your ultrasound be familiar with using the test to help diagnose the condition.

Diet and Lifestyle Change

Medications can help level the hormonal playing field, but they can only take you so far. Learning how to eat and be active in a way that treats the underlying insulin resistance in PCOS is key to improving fertility, reducing the risk of diabetes (both type 2 and gestational), and lowering your risk of life-threatening cardiovascular complications. Step one is to convince yourself you can do it. This can be a tough personal sell if you've struggled with your diet and weight for ages. But there is no sense wasting time torturing yourself over all the things you think you've done wrong in the past. You can't rewrite history, but you can learn from it. Take stock of what helped you change your diet, add in exercise, or lose weight in the past—as well as what didn't help. What's left is an honest assessment of where your strengths arc and what you need to work on to evolve your diet and lifestyle habits to a healthier place. Emphasize the positive steps you can take to make change; focus on the foods and activities you can *add* to your life, not the things you think you can't have or can't do.

Healthy eating means going out of your way to eat good, nourishing food—not hyperfocusing on all the "bad food" you need to avoid. I'm a big believer in embracing the 80/20 rule. Assume that roughly 80 percent of what you eat and how active you are represents your habits, and that roughly 20 percent of the time your day won't go as usual—you'll have to wing it, sometimes not resulting in the best choices. At first you may allow for a once-a-week indulgence just because you like it, it feels good, or you just want to let go and enjoy something. Or you may feel comfortable setting the bar a little higher, preferring a 90/10 approach. The idea is that you have to make space in your diet and lifestyle for special treats and indulgences, without expecting perfection. Your habits affect your health, and in our culture these habits often need a major league overhaul.

The 80/20 approach—even the 90/10 approach—allows for us to be imperfect dieters, something the country's dieting history has not allowed

Mind-Set Intervention: Finding Support

No one ever makes revolutionary changes in her life (or in the lives of others) by operating from a position of self-defeat. If you need therapy to help get beyond the negative or destructive thinking, find a therapist with expertise in your issue and go for it! Don't shy away from this kind of help if you need it. You need to throw the book at PCOS, and much of what it takes to change starts between your ears! If it's a food or body issue, find a therapist passionate and experienced in those issues. You deserve someone who's going to embrace your issues. For leads on who these folks might be in your community, search local eating-disorder support organizations, which usually include help for compulsive overeating.

for. Historically, certain words have defined how virtuous we are about losing weight, and they're loaded with judgment: "being good," "sticking to the plan," "I haven't cheated," "I don't do that anymore." We're just as good at dressing ourselves down: "I was bad," "I cheated," "I fell off the plan," "I was good for a while but then I lost it." Let's be clear: human beings are not perfect. We make mistakes. In fact, we usually need to make mistakes to learn how to change. It's kind of like the difference between being told about something new versus researching it yourself—actually looking it up and reading about it. Maybe even writing about it. The more you delve into the new information, the more it has a chance to sink in and become a part of you.

. . .

It may be hard work, but permanent change comes from hard work, and diets don't often demand that of us in the long term. This is particularly true of weight loss programs where you buy all your food from the plan. What's going to happen when you decide you don't want to live for the rest of your life on prepackaged microwave meals? But that's not to say you can't learn something from these plans (or haven't in the past) that could end up being an important part of your own personalized portfolio plan of skills and habits that finally work long term for you. For many people, past dieting experiences offer important hints about what helps (and doesn't help) you set the stage for the kind of eating and activity habits you want to adopt.

2

An Internal Look at PCOS

An important part of understanding how to manage your polycystic ovary syndrome is to truly understand what's going on in your body and how what you do affects it. Your goal should be to manage your PCOS as naturally as possible so that you're only relying on medications to fill the gap between the progress you make with diet and activity. My experience has shown me that most women with PCOS don't really understand their condition. They read a lot of information on the Internet or in books but have trouble internalizing how making changes in their diet and activity patterns will affect how they feel in their body every day. This is particularly true for women who have come to view their body as the enemy and think that only major weight loss will make them feel better. Getting PCOS symptoms under control can help a woman see the light at the end of the tunnel. If you're not moody and craving carbs all the time, you may just start to believe that change is possible! First you have to understand what's going on inside and how your lifestyle habits may make it better or worse.

Understanding Insulin Resistance

As far back as the early 1900s, a reference was made in a French medical article by Archard and Theirs to "bearded lady diabetes," marking the first clinical connection between PCOS and the function of the hormone insulin.[1] Despite this earlier observation, as well as subsequent research illuminating the effects that insulin has on the ovaries, addressing insulin resistance as the root cause in the majority of PCOS cases didn't come about until relatively recently. Reproductive endocrinologist Dr. Jeffrey Chang published a report linking PCOS with insulin resistance in the early 1980s, and prolific PCOS researcher Dr. Andrea Dunaif published clinical studies on PCOS and insulin resistance in 1989.[2] Since that time, major strides have been made clarifying the connection between insulin resistance and PCOS, but the area continues to evolve.[3] Much of our understanding of how treating insulin resistance could affect fertility initially came from pharmaceutical studies on diabetes drugs that found they were affecting weight, menstrual cycle length, and fertility. This led to off-label clinical use of insulin-altering drugs to treat PCOS, which has since become mainstream in treating the fertility effects of the disorder and reducing the risk of diabetes. But what exactly is insulin resistance, and what can be done about it?

Insulin is a protein made up of a long chain of amino acids (little protein units) and is produced in the beta cells of the pancreas. Like other hormones in the body, insulin is released into the blood to travel around the body, exerting its effect. Insulin's major action is to dictate how the body uses energy. Glucose is the body's main fuel and energy source, and its presence in the blood stimulates insulin's release into circulation. In return, insulin secretion is critical to maintaining a stable and steady supply of glucose to the cells. Generally speaking, the secretion of insulin is regulated to keep blood glucose levels between 70 and 115 milligrams per deciliter (mg/dl); the number may vary some between laboratories. If blood glucose levels drop too low, this is called *hypoglycemia*. If someone is hypoglycemic, they may start out feeling a little "fuzzy," like they're not thinking as clearly as usual, and hungry—often for the carbohydrates the body uses to replenish its blood glucose supply. If hypoglycemia progresses to dangerously low levels, which would only happen to a diabetic who has taken too much injectable insulin, unconsciousness can result and possibly even death. In *hyperglycemia*, or high blood glucose, the body tries to produce as much excess insulin as it can in an effort to lower blood glucose levels, but if it can't this eventually results in diabetes. The body attempts to rid itself of excess glucose by urinating it out through the kidneys (this accounts for the frequent urination and subsequent thirst seen as a symptom of diabetes).

At times when energy in the form of food exceeds what the body needs, insulin will promote the storage of glucose in the liver and muscle as glycogen, which is basically little sugar cubes of glucose stored for later use as fuel. When these reserves are filled, additional excess glucose is stored as body fat, an important calorie reserve that was critical to survival throughout most of human history, when food supplies where much more variable.

Insulin not only promotes the storage of glucose as fat and glycogen but also interferes with the breakdown of body fat (lipolysis) and glycogen (glycogenolysis) to be used as fuel. We humans still have the same genes as those who lived during the Stone Age, and in many parts of the world even today, human beings are at chronic risk of starving to death. During conditions of drought or famine, it was good if insulin worked hard to encourage the storage of calorie reserves, making sure any withdrawn calories were being put to good use before letting them go. But in this day and age, this same once protective mechanism is backfiring, making it tough for us to shed excess calorie reserves that can become a health liability. As with many modern-day health problems, it's a bit of "good gene gone bad"—what was helpful in an evolutionary sense is now harmful. Like many hormones, this critical role insulin plays as an energy regulator is just one of its many roles. Insulin has many "target tissues" or cells throughout the body that rely on it for lots of important functions. The liver, muscles, blood vessels, the pituitary gland, and the brain all interact with insulin to perform different metabolic actions. Some of these effects may play an as-yet not fully understood role in the pathophysiology of PCOS. What follows is a basic description of the complex action of insulin. The goal is to help you understand in simple terms the essence of what goes on so you can visualize how what (and how) you eat affects your glucose-insulin response.

To facilitate the clearance of sugar out of the blood and into the cells, where it can be used for fuel, insulin acts like a key, connecting with a special lock on the cells called an insulin receptor. Once the insulin locates an insulin receptor on the cell, the insulin will connect with it and, in essence, unlock the cell, allowing glucose to travel out of the blood and into the cell to be used as fuel. This complex process involves a series of events all geared toward allowing the cell access to an energy source. Under normal circumstances the insulin receptors are sufficiently sensitive to the action of insulin to allow the cell to be opened using "normal" amounts of insulin. But some people don't use insulin as effectively as they should, a condition called insulin resistance (IR), which makes their cells less sensitive to the action of insulin. In other words, the insulin comes knocking on the cell door, but the cell won't unlock the door. The connection just isn't right. The pancreas will sense this is going on and respond to this resistance by secreting more insulin into the blood, the goal of which is to overwhelm the cell with enough additional insulin that it will "force" the glucose into the cell.

The result? Glucose clears out of the blood and into the cell, but at the expense of making the pancreas work harder than it should have to. If this goes unchecked (or untreated by diet, exercise, and medications if needed) over time, this can exhaust the pancreas, rendering it less able to produce insulin. When the pancreas no longer has the reserves to oversecrete insulin in response to IR, glucose will cease to fully clear out of the blood, which initially shows up as impaired glucose tolerance on a fasting glucose test and often eventually diabetes.[4] Because you can't rebuild the pancreas's ability to produce insulin (you can only learn how to work with it as a lifelong limitation), once you have diabetes, you cannot cure it; you can only manage it. In the case of insulin resistance, an ounce of prevention is clearly worth a pound of cure—it's much easier to prevent diabetes from happening than to take care of it once it occurs.

Once this excess insulin is secreted into the blood, it stands to negatively affect the many other functions of the body that are also influenced by insulin. What we now know about PCOS is that while some tissues can be resistant to the action of insulin (mostly muscle cells, which gobble up 30 percent of the calories we eat), other cells remain sensitive to it, including the ovaries. When an ovary is overexposed to insulin, it increases its production of androgens (male-type hormones), which accounts for many of the signs and symptoms of PCOS.

An Inherited Trait

Insulin resistance is a strongly inherited trait—if others in your family have PCOS, metabolic syndrome, prediabetes, or diabetes, your chances of having it as well are increased. But IR is hardly black or white. There is great variability in how sensitively an individual processes insulin, much of which would fall within the normal range. Historically, insulin resistance was a good thing. It protected us from the effects of starvation. Muscle cells are big consumers of glucose. They need it to sustain activity, which was particularly important when human beings expended a lot of energy hunting and gathering food. But the central nervous system needs glucose too—to the tune of about four hundred to six hundred glucose calories a day to fuel your brain, spinal column, and nervous system.[5] If under conditions of physiological stress, as would be experienced during conditions of drought or famine, our muscle cells gobbled up the bulk of any incoming glucose, the nervous system wouldn't get its fair share. Making the muscle cells somewhat resistant to the action of insulin during periods of physiological stress would help preserve some glucose in the blood for your brain and other nervous system tissues. But what was once good is now not so good for many people. Today, overnourishment and inactivity, and their accompanying physiological side effects, have created a harmful condition in many of us.

Insulin resistance has a long genetic history and is strongly affected by diet, weight, activity, and lifestyle. If you have a genetic predisposition to

Common Complaints Related to Insulin Resistance

How do you know if you have insulin resistance? Beyond using blood tests to reveal IR, there aren't any universal signs and symptoms. However, many people with IR have similar complaints that may be related to IR. They include the following:

- Fluctuations in energy level throughout the day—some women start off energetic but crash in the afternoon.
- Frequent hunger, and after they've eaten, these women don't feel full for long.
- Binge eating at meals.
- Constant cravings for sweets and other refined (white) carbohydrates, like white bread, crackers, or pasta. Not uncommonly, those with IR describe feeling "addicted to sweets" and feel they can't be trusted around them!
- Irritability if they go too long without eating, which might not be long at all compared to people without IR.
- Severe intolerance to low-calorie diets, particularly those that severely limit carbohydrates.

Obviously, these signs and symptoms can occur and still be totally unrelated to IR, but in my practice these are commonly expressed complaints. What's striking about many women with PCOS is a feeling that food has an unusual hold over them that they don't think most people have. They describe a feeling of being "addicted" to carbohydrates. It's not surprising that binge eating, or compulsive overeating, is common in women with PCOS.

IR, it has a much greater chance of expressing itself if you're overweight and sedentary. There are many people with insulin resistance and diabetes who would not have it if they were at a healthy weight and led an active lifestyle. At the same time there are many normal-range-weight, active people who would be insulin resistant and possibly diabetic if they were overweight and sedentary.

It's hard to say exactly how many people in the United States have insulin resistance because it is frequently undiagnosed until it turns into prediabetes or diabetes. We do have striking numbers on these two conditions, however. According to the Centers for Disease Control (CDC), about *fifty-four million* individuals in the United States ages twenty-one and older have prediabetes. Data from 2007 show that approximately twenty-four million Americans have diabetes, or roughly 8 percent of the population (six million of whom don't know they have it). In the United States approximately one of every three persons born in 2000 will develop diabetes in his or her lifetime. The lifetime risk of developing diabetes is even greater for ethnic minorities, where two of every five African-Americans and Hispanics (one of every two Hispanic *females*) will develop the disease.

As scary as all this is, not all the news is bad. According to the CDC, progression to diabetes among those with prediabetes is *not* inevitable. Studies show that people with prediabetes who lose at least 7 percent of their body weight and engage in moderate physical activity at least 150 minutes a week can prevent or delay diabetes and even return their blood glucose levels to normal. Research shows that intensive lifestyle interventions are the most effective way to prevent or delay type 2 diabetes.[6] Other studies have looked at insulin sensitivity in healthy individuals, where there was 600 percent variability in how sensitively their study subjects used insulin—ranging from the most insulin sensitive to the least. The author of this study estimated that about 25 percent of that variability is probably due to being overweight, 25 percent is related to fitness level, with the remaining 50 percent possibly genetic.[7] This suggests there is potentially a lot of room for positively influencing any genetic predisposition to diabetes with diet and lifestyle change.

Insulin Resistance and the Ovaries

Let's look at what happens during normal ovulation. Women are born with all the eggs in our ovaries we're ever going to have (somewhere in the neighborhood of two million, which is reduced into the thousands by the time a young woman starts ovulating). Generally, one at a time (or more in the case of fraternal twins), the eggs get in line to undergo hormonally induced changes that ready them for ovulation and fertilization. Four major hormones are involved in maturing eggs: follicle stimulating hormone (FSH) and luteinizing hormone (LH) are called gonadotropins and are released from the pituitary gland in the brain; estradiol and progesterone are steroids (sex hormones) and are secreted by the ovary. FSH and estrogen are involved in the follicular phase of egg maturation, which runs from the onset of your period until ovulation, and LH and progesterone are involved in the luteal phase, which occurs from the time between ovulation and your next period.

In a normal menstrual cycle FSH from the pituitary stimulates egg follicles to develop, stimulating estrogen production in the ovary, which in turn stimulates the release of LH from the pituitary. LH then triggers ovulation (the release of a mature egg from the ovary into the fallopian tube, where it can be fertilized by a sperm) and stimulates progesterone production in the ovary, which prepares the body for pregnancy. It's basically a hormonal ping-pong game between your pituitary and your ovaries. If all goes as planned, an egg is released, ripe and ready for fertilization. If fertilization doesn't occur, progesterone levels drop, the lining of the uterus is shed, and the cycle starts over again.

There is still a lot we don't know about PCOS. The syndrome is extremely complicated and occurs with varying degrees of severity. These hormones mentioned are just part of what determines whether conception occurs or not. It has been known that a relationship exists between insulin and ovarian androgen production for more than twenty-five years. Although much has yet to be learned about the complex hormonal effects of PCOS, several different effects are believed to possibly occur when an ovary is overexposed to insulin:

• Increased testosterone production.
• Increased luteinizing hormone (LH) production.

- Decreased production of sex hormone binding globulin (SHBG), a substance that binds to hormones, making them less able to exert their effect in the blood.
- Interaction with leptin, a hormone that triggers satiety, or a sense of fullness.
- Interruption of normal ovulation.[8]

Luteinizing hormone and insulin primarily regulate androgen production in the ovary. The gonadotropin LH is secreted by the pituitary gland (which also regulates the thyroid and adrenal glands); insulin is secreted by the pancreas. Both insulin and LH can stimulate androgen production, but how they relate to each other differs—elevated levels of insulin can raise your LH levels, but high levels of LH don't raise insulin levels. Having elevations in both insulin and LH is considered a sign of more serious PCOS. A common finding in PCOS is elevated levels of LH. LH acts to stimulate the theca cells in the ovary (the layer of cells surrounding the follicle) to produce androgens. It is thought that higher levels of LH can stimulate excess androgen production, blocking the follicles from further development, ultimately leading to their demise.

In addition to hormones, numerous enzymes, growth factors, and other chemicals are involved in the exquisite hormonal regulation that occurs within what's called the "hypothalamic-pituitary-ovarian axis" that regulates reproduction, many of which could somehow be involved in the abnormalities seen in women with PCOS. The reproductive aspects of PCOS can be boiled down to several facts: PCOS is tied to abnormal hormonal signaling from the ovaries that interferes with the normal maturation and ovulation of eggs in the ovaries. The stage at which the follicles generally stop developing normally is the testosterone-producing phase, resulting in higher levels of testosterone than estrogen, creating an environment where testosterone's effects are dominating. The hormonal problems that arise in the ovaries have a trickle-down (or out!) effect that spreads around the body, producing the far-reaching signs and symptoms of PCOS, and the severity of any of these effects can vary between women.

PCOS and Your Heart

Women with PCOS are among one of the highest-risk groups for cardio-vascular disease. Studies show that starting at a younger age, women with PCOS tend to have higher LDL, lower HDL, and higher triglycerides (blood fats) than women without PCOS, which could result in earlier onset of cardiovascular disease. The insulin resistance seen in women with PCOS can affect nitric oxide function in the endothelium (inner lining) of the blood vessels. This makes them less malleable, or less able to dilate as needed to accommodate blood flow, which over time can increase the risk for cardiovascular disease. One study showed that 12 percent of women with PCOS have hypertension, although this is more common in women who are overweight. The syndrome has been tied to two blood markers that may suggest an increased risk of heart disease: (1) higher levels of plasminogen activator inhibitor-1 (also called PAI-1), which is an inhibitor of fibrinolysis, the physiological process that breaks down blood clots; and (2) higher levels of C-reactive protein, an indicator of inflammation. Insulin resistance, diabetes, and abdominal obesity—all potentially present in PCOS—are risk factors for heart disease.[9]

Interestingly, there are a few studies that don't show an increased risk of cardiovascular disease in women with PCOS. This may reflect the notion that there is something in some women with PCOS that protects them from increased risk. There's also the fact that being overweight or obese—for women with or without PCOS—will increase the risk of heart disease, as will any number of individual risk factors found in women with PCOS (high cholesterol, high blood pressure, and so on). More long-term research is needed to further explore the cardiovascular-PCOS connection.

PCOS versus Metabolic Syndrome

In many ways the risk factors seen in women with PCOS are the same as those seen in people who have metabolic syndrome, a condition known to be a preemptor of heart disease and diabetes.[10] This syndrome is characterized by a group of metabolic risk factors that include abdominal obesity (excessive fat in and around the abdomen); abnormal blood cholesterol and fat (lipid) disorders—high triglycerides, low HDL cholesterol, and high LDL cholesterol—that encourage plaque buildup in artery walls; elevated blood pressure; insulin resistance or glucose intolerance (indicating prediabetes); prothrombotic state, or a difficulty breaking down blood clots (more specifically, high fibrinogen or plasminogen activator inhibitor-1 in the blood); and proinflammatory state (elevated levels of C-reactive protein in the blood, an indicator of inflammation in the body).

Many of these same factors are criteria used to determine whether a woman has PCOS. In fact, it's estimated that about 50 percent or more of women with PCOS meet the criteria for metabolic syndrome, which is becoming increasingly common and is believed to affect more than fifty million men and women in the United States. But metabolic syndrome affects both men *and* women, and clearly not every woman with metabolic syndrome has PCOS. Like PCOS, as a syndrome a diagnosis of metabolic syndrome is arrived at by determining whether someone's clinical picture meets enough diagnostic criteria. According to the American Heart Association and the National Heart, Lung, and Blood Institute, metabolic syndrome is identified with the presence of three or more of these components:

- Elevated waist circumference: for men, equal to or greater than 40 inches (102 cm); for women, equal to or greater than 35 inches (88 cm)
- Elevated triglycerides: equal to or greater than 150 mg/dl
- Reduced HDL cholesterol: for men, less than 40 mg/dl; for women, less than 50 mg/dl
- Elevated blood pressure: equal to or greater than 130/85 mm Hg
- Elevated fasting glucose: equal to or greater than 100 mg/dl

Given the major crossover of PCOS and metabolic syndrome, the treatment of cardiovascular risk in both conditions is the same: weight loss through diet change and increased activity, and control of individual metabolic risk factors (high blood pressure, abnormal blood lipids, prediabetes) through diet and lifestyle change (and medications as needed). And there's a significant trickle-down effect: anything you do to improve your cardiovascular health will benefit your overall health in many ways, including reducing your risk of cancer, keeping your brain sharp, and trimming your waistline!

The Emotional Influence of PCOS

Numerous studies have suggested a connection between PCOS and such emotional disorders as depression, anxiety, body image issues, and eating disorders.[11] Given the issues surrounding PCOS for many women, this shouldn't be surprising. What's hard to tease out is how much of what is affecting a woman's emotional health is related specifically to the condition (hormones or blood glucose fluctuations perhaps) or the other baggage that tends to come along with PCOS (weight struggles, fears about one's health, body image anxiety due to weight, excess hair growth, hair loss, acne, and so on). Layer onto that the relentless stress of infertility for some women, and emotional distress is easy to understand. It's important to seek help from a qualified therapist or support group when you need it (see chapter 13 for more on this).

· · ·

If you have PCOS, it's easy to feel like you're drowning in the details. Delving too much into the realities of the syndrome can be at a minimum discouraging and at worst paralyzing. It's most helpful to focus on what can be done based on what is known about the syndrome scientifically. When it comes to managing your PCOS, knowledge is power—understanding what is going on and developing an action plan can help you feel more in control. With this knowledge, you'll feel more optimistic that you can take charge of your health.

3

Treating PCOS: Diet, Nutrition, and Medication

As you learn the ins and outs of polycystic ovary syndrome, it might be tempting to consider whether there is a medication that can just make it go away. If only it were this easy. Treating PCOS may require additional help from medications, but like many chronic conditions, diet and lifestyle change should be your priority. Once you've determined how far you can manage the condition with diet and lifestyle changes, you may then get an additional leg up from medications that may help you meet your goals of losing weight, lowering your risk of diabetes, managing your symptoms, and improving your fertility (if that's on your list). But medications will only get you so far. Just like using them to help manage other chronic health problems—including obesity, diabetes, heart disease, some forms of arthritis, and so on—most ailments benefit from a natural approach as well, and medications won't compensate for a bad diet or lack of regular activity. Plus, medications are usually expensive. With the state of today's health-care system, who knows what insurance will (or won't) cover in the future?

As with many people suffering from a chronic health problem, women with PCOS often feel unwell and dissatisfied with their bodies. They may have spent years trying to get a diagnosis, seeing countless doctors to have their symptoms treated, but never really getting to the root of the problem. For their irregular periods, they've been put on birth control pills. They might have used electrolysis to deal with unsightly facial hair. Thinning hair on the head? Try Rogaine or some other "alternative" treatment of questionable benefit. High cholesterol? They've been told to change their diet and maybe consider cholesterol-lowering medication. Acne? See a dermatologist. Feeling frustrated and depressed? Think about therapy. The list of potential solutions for these and other symptoms of PCOS goes on and on, many of which may have proven somewhat helpful. Some of these solutions may have served as temporary fixes; others may have ultimately led to complete dead ends. It's possible that some of these treatments would have provided even more relief if there had been accompanying diet and lifestyle changes.

Although many women are extremely grateful to finally be told that what they're feeling isn't all in their heads, they're often overwhelmed by what it will take to heal themselves. Because of the underlying insulin resistance seen in most cases of PCOS—and the accompanying increased risk of diabetes and heart disease—the syndrome requires significant diet and lifestyle change, possibly in combination with medication. Being told to lose weight and change your diet one more time, without really understanding exactly *why* it will make a difference, can bring even the most determined woman to tears. It's natural to experience mixed emotions when you finally find out you have PCOS, particularly if you're also in the throes of a fertility workup or some other stressful life event. But understand this: PCOS is treatable. It is not a terminal disease with few treatment options. You can gain control over your health in many ways that are not much different than what everyone should be doing to live long, healthy lives. The key to truly taking control of this syndrome is to really understand what PCOS is, how it affects your body functions, and how its many aspects can be treated so you can just get on with your life!

Making a Difference with Diet and Lifestyle

Scientists, physicians, and nutritionists are in the early stages of trying to understand the best diet and lifestyle strategies for women with PCOS. It would be ideal to have the results of a number of large-scale studies on what kinds of diet and lifestyle habits are most beneficial—and why. But until that day comes, the best bet is to follow our hunches based on research to date and clinical experience. We know how to help people lose weight. We know how to improve blood cholesterol levels and control high blood pressure. We know that exercise is critical to reducing the risk of just about every chronic disease you can think of. And we have some good leads on diet and lifestyle strategies that will likely help a large percentage of women with PCOS. The research points to several promising areas.

A 2007 study from the University of California–Davis of twenty-eight women with PCOS looked at the relationship between nutrients and hormones known to be clinically important in this condition. The women in the study ate their usual diet and then drank either seventy-five grams of glucose (sugar) or seventy-five grams of whey protein in liquid form. Blood levels of several hormones in the women were tested five hours later. The results showed significantly higher blood glucose and insulin levels in the hours after the glucose drink. Hyperinsulinemia (high insulin levels), which contributes to obesity by encouraging fatty acids to deposit into the body fat while also inhibiting its release from fat stores, also aggravates hormones known to be part of PCOS. Two-thirds of the patients with PCOS had hypoglycemia after drinking the glucose drink; they also experienced greater increases in their cortisol and DHEA levels (another hormone often elevated in PCOS). The stress hormone cortisol can contribute to obesity by increasing hunger and cravings for sweets and fatty foods and encouraging the deposit of fat in the abdomen. It also stimulates the release of glucose from the liver—raising blood glucose levels—and aggravates insulin resistance. Even more interestingly, the glucose drink suppressed levels of ghrelin, often referred to as "the hunger hormone," for shorter periods of time than the protein drink. This means that it took longer for the subjects to feel hungry after the protein drink. Although this study used protein and glucose drinks as opposed to foods high in protein and carbs, these findings support the potential benefit of including a higher amount of protein in the diet for women with PCOS.[1]

A 2009 study from the University of California–Davis compared the effects of protein versus simple sugar on weight loss, body composition, and blood levels of fasting glucose, insulin, and cholesterol levels in twenty-four women with PCOS. Researchers first decreased the diet by 700 calories overall and then added back a 250-calorie supplement of either whey protein or simple sugar, so the overall calorie reduction was 450 calories fewer per day. The results? The protein-supplemented subjects lost more weight and more body fat, had larger decreases in total cholesterol, and higher levels of healthy HDL. This study provides support for the potential benefits of including more protein and limiting added sugars.[2]

A 2004 study from Pennsylvania State University's Department of Obstetrics and Gynecology divided thirty-five obese women with PCOS into two calorie-restricted groups: one a high-protein group (30 percent protein, 40 percent carbohydrate, 30 percent fat) and one a high-carbohydrate group (15 percent protein, 55 percent carbohydrate, 30 percent fat). Twenty-six of the women completed the study. After one month on the diets both groups lost a significant amount of weight (an average of four pounds in each group), with no significant differences between the two groups. Both groups experienced improvements in their circulating androgen levels, fasting insulin levels, and three-hour glucose tolerance tests. This study supports the belief that even modest weight loss can improve circulating levels of hormones and improve insulin sensitivity, regardless of how the calorie reduction is achieved. It was, however, a very short-term study, so it doesn't tell us much about how to achieve a lasting calorie reduction.[3]

A 2005 weight-loss study from the University of Colorado looked at the calorie composition question a little differently. The researchers did not look at women with PCOS specifically; rather, they studied obese nondiabetic women who had been determined to be either insulin sensitive or insulin resistant. Again, this was a fairly small study of only twenty-one women ages twenty-three to fifty-three. In both the insulin-sensitive and insulin-resistant groups, women were put on either a high-carb (60 percent) and low-fat (20 percent) diet or a low-carb (40 percent) and high-fat (40 percent) diet; both groups were calorie restricted to promote weight loss. Interestingly, in this study what type of diet resulted in more weight loss depended on whether the woman showed signs of insulin resistance. Over the sixteen weeks of the study, the insulin-sensitive women lost more weight on the high-carb diet, and the insulin-resistant women lost more weight on the low-carb diet. Both groups lost an average of about 13.5 pounds. Given that most women with PCOS are assumed to have some degree of insulin resistance, this study supports moderating carbohydrate intake. It's important to keep in mind that these were calorie-restricted diets, so even the diet that allowed more fat would have capped the total amount of fat one could consume. And the "low-carb" diet in this study wasn't anywhere near as low in carbohydrates as many recent popular low-carb weight-loss diets.[4]

Weight Loss and Fertility

Because problems with fertility are so common in women with PCOS, a significant body of research has analyzed the various connections between diet, exercise, weight loss, and fertility. A 2003 study from the University of Adelaide in Australia looked at the effect of diet composition in forty-five women with PCOS. Women were counseled on a calorie-restricted diet for weight loss that was either 55 percent carb, 15 percent protein, and 30 percent fat (which they referred to as the "low-protein diet") or 40 percent carb, 30 percent protein, and 30 percent fat (which was considered their "high-protein" intervention). The weight-loss phase of the diet was twelve weeks, followed by a four-week maintenance phase. The subjects were advised to exercise a minimum of three times a week.

The major findings of the Adelaide study were that both groups had lost weight—an average of 15 pounds in the low-protein group and 18.7 pounds in the high-protein group. Both groups also experienced an on-average 20 percent drop in fasting insulin in the weight-loss phase that they were able to maintain in the weight-maintenance phase, and 44 percent had an improvement in their ovulation. Three pregnancies also occurred—one on the low-protein diet and two on the high-protein diet—with an approximate conception time at about four to five weeks on the diet after an

Insulin Resistance and Fertility

What does any of this have to do with the ovaries? When it comes to clearing sugars out of the blood, the primary targets for insulin are the muscles, the liver, and fatty tissues. So in insulin-resistant people the pancreas is secreting excess insulin primarily to overcome insulin resistance in these tissues. But other tissues throughout the body are not insulin resistant. In fact, many are quite sensitive to insulin, including the ovaries. Some researchers think the ovaries of women with PCOS may be uniquely influenced by insulin in a way that is not yet fully understood. When ovaries are overexposed to insulin, they increase their production of androgens (like testosterone), which interferes with the action of several other hormones and ultimately can upset the very delicate hormonal balance that must occur to ready eggs for ovulation and fertilization.

average 11- to 12-pound weight loss. The subjects on the high-protein diet experienced somewhat better improvements in their cholesterol profiles and reproductive function. Although this study was too small to draw firm conclusions, it seems to again support the benefits of even modest weight loss at improving the health and fertility of women with PCOS.[5]

A 2003 study from the University of Milan in Italy of thirty-three overweight women with PCOS who either didn't ovulate or ovulated infrequently found that a 1200-calorie restricted diet and regular exercise had a significant effect on their rates of ovulation. Twenty-five of the thirty-three patients lost at least 5 percent of their weight; eleven patients (33 percent) lost at least 10 percent of their weight. Regular menstrual cycles returned in 72 percent of the patients who complied with the diet, and of the women who lost at least 5 percent of their weight, 40 percent subsequently became pregnant.[6]

These most recent studies on diet and PCOS have been fairly small, so the optimal dietary treatment for the syndrome is not yet clear. Large-scale studies could offer some important insights into the most effective diet for women with PCOS, but for now our best bet is to avoid any extreme approaches that could inflict potential harm. Studies so far strongly support that eating well and exercising regularly can make a major difference. We do know that weight loss via any approach will benefit PCOS, from both an overall health and fertility standpoint. Weight loss decreases insulin resistance, blood androgen levels, ovary size, and the number of ovarian cysts, and enhances fertility. It also improves blood cholesterol levels, lowering "bad" cholesterol and boosting "good" cholesterol. Some research supports the usefulness of a higher-protein diet (as opposed to high carb), because of its ties to longer satiety (fullness), maintenance of muscle mass, weight maintenance, and healthy cholesterol levels.

Diet and Insulin Resistance

Insulin resistance is an amazingly complex condition associated with a host of different health problems besides PCOS, including diabetes, gestational diabetes, metabolic syndrome, cardiovascular disease, fatty liver, and several different types of cancer. But don't despair! Controlling insulin resistance will trickle down to lowering the risks of any of these diseases.

Let's start by looking at some facts about glucose. Glucose, or blood sugar, is the primary source of fuel for the human body, feeding all of the body's cells, including muscles, organs (like the liver and brain), and body fat. There has to be some sugar in the blood at all times or you wouldn't be alive. A normal blood sugar generally runs somewhere between 70 and 115 milligrams per deciliter (mg/dl). The sugar that's in our blood is a combination of sugars released from glucose reserves in the liver, called glycogen, and sugars released into the blood after the digestion of food, mainly dietary carbohydrates. When you eat carbohydrates, it takes about an hour for the majority of the carbs to be digested down to their most basic units—sugars—and released into your blood.

How rapidly those sugars arrive in your blood depends on how easy it is to digest the carb that you ate. In general, the more refined or processed a carbohydrate is before you eat it, the less work your body has to do on the inside to finish up the digestion process and release the sugars into the blood. For example, soda is already liquid sugar, so it will be released into your blood as glucose faster than the sugars from a bowl of plain, whole grain oatmeal, which is eaten much closer to its natural state. The rate of carbohydrate breakdown—and therefore how rapidly your blood glucose levels will rise after eating a carb—can be influenced by the glycemic index or the glycemic load of a food (see chapter 4 for more on this). How much sugar will ultimately be released into your blood is directly related to how much carbohydrate you ate—a large portion will result in a larger infusion of glucose into the blood than a smaller portion.

Now, with the basics of blood sugar in hand, let's review blood sugar processing, using the experience of an imaginary, non-insulin-resistant woman, Marie. Here's the stripped-down version of the blood sugar–insulin relationship:

1. Marie hasn't eaten in a while, so she has a normal, baseline amount of sugar circulating in her blood.
2. Time for lunch! Marie sits down and eats a turkey sandwich, a glass of milk, and an orange. The bread from the sandwich, the milk, and the orange all contain carbohydrates.
3. Within an hour of eating, the majority of the carbs Marie ate at lunchtime have been broken down and are showing up as sugar in

her blood. She now has her baseline blood sugars plus the sugars from the carbs she ate an hour ago.

4. The excess sugars from the foods Marie just digested don't want to linger in her blood for long. They want to move out of her blood and enter her cells all around her body, so the cells can be energized and Marie's blood sugar can return to normal. But the sugars in her blood can't just "float" out of her blood and into her cells. In order for the sugar to enter the cells, the cells need to be "unlocked" with the help of insulin, a hormone produced by the pancreas. The pancreas hangs off the digestive tract, close to where the sugars exit the intestine and enter the bloodstream. (Besides being involved in sugar metabolism, the pancreas also secretes digestive enzymes into the intestine to help break down food into nutrients.) Shortly after the sugar shows up in the blood, the blood with the sugar in it will circulate through the pancreas, which will detect the presence of sugar in the blood. In response to this, the pancreas secretes insulin into the bloodstream.

5. Now Marie has insulin circulating in her blood, along with glucose. Think of insulin as a bunch of little keys that rush around the body, unlocking the cells so sugars can exit the blood and enter the cells to be incinerated for energy.

6. For the insulin keys to unlock the cells, they must first connect with keyholes on the cells called insulin receptors. Once the insulin and insulin receptors connect, the cells open up and allow the sugar to enter. This whole process takes about two hours, at which point Marie's blood sugar should be back within a normal range.

How is this blood sugar–insulin relationship different if someone has insulin resistance? Let's take a look at Paula, our imaginary insulin-resistant woman with PCOS:

1. Paula just had lunch with Marie and ate the same thing—including the carbs from the bread, milk, and fruit.

2. Like Marie, Paula's pancreas got the message about sugar in the blood and released what it thought should be the amount of insulin necessary to unlock the cells and clear the excess sugars out of the blood. In her case, however, things don't go exactly as they should.

3. When the insulin from Paula's pancreas approaches the cells to hook up with a receptor, the insulin and receptor don't connect as efficiently as they should. The insulin is knocking on the cell door, but the cell is holding the door shut! The pancreas senses that this is happening—the sugars just aren't clearing out of the blood as efficiently as they should—and responds by secreting more insulin out into the blood, with the idea of overwhelming the cells with extra insulin: in effect, forcing the cells open.

The pancreas is pretty good at doing this, because the sugars do eventually clear out of the blood. The problem is that over time this need to work in overdrive can exhaust the pancreas to the point where it's no longer able to secrete enough extra insulin to overcome insulin resistance. Hence the increased risk for diabetes in anyone with insulin resistance. The pancreas may eventually wear out from overuse.

As mentioned, there are some women with PCOS who do not appear to be insulin resistant, and others who are insulin resistant but don't have PCOS. Going with the best information available, the primary treatment goal of PCOS is to lower circulating insulin levels. For many women that involves significant dietary change, increased exercise, and possibly medication, to manage their health and hormones. The primary treatment for this syndrome is thus diet and exercise, augmented with medication if necessary, particularly if you're looking to enhance your fertility. Drugs simply can't compensate for the damage an unhealthy lifestyle can inflict.

Why Diet Makes a Difference

Subsequent chapters offer detailed advice on exactly how to eat to lower insulin levels, but here we look at why diet makes a difference, using our insulin-resistant friend Paula. Compared to Marie, who is easily able to mobilize sugars out of her blood after eating, Paula has a handicap in that her insulin is not used as efficiently. Like anyone with a physical challenge, it may seem tough at first, but Paula's best bet is to learn to work with her challenge. This means doing what she can to take the pressure off her pancreas, so it doesn't feel the need to work so hard, and taking advantage of natural means of sensitizing her cells to the action of insulin.

Once you eat carbs, within an hour your blood is flooded with sugar, the end products of carbohydrate digestion. The presence of sugar in the blood stimulates the pancreas to secrete insulin. And blood sugar and insulin have a linear relationship—the more sugar in the blood, the more aggressive the insulin response. But the reverse is also true: the lighter the sugar load, the less the insulin response. This is a critical player in taking pressure off the pancreas. Think about it: what dictates how hard your pancreas has to work? The amount of sugar in the blood. What dictates that? The amount of carbohydrates you ate an hour ago. So if the goal is to lessen your insulin response, you need to spread your carbs out more over the day in smaller portions, focusing on less processed, more nutritious carbohydrates. This is the foundation of the PCOS diet plan, what I call the carbohydrate-distributed diet. Not too high in carbs, but not so low that you miss out on many of the well-established health benefits of including good-quality carbs in the diet.

To illustrate the carb-distributed diet, let's look at two sample daily meal patterns: (1) three large meals a day and (2) three smaller meals plus two snacks a day. First, let's look at the three-large-meal pattern.

In this first example the day's foods are basically broken down into three meals. Food intake data tells us that the average American diet is about 50 percent carbohydrate, so let's assume each of these three meals is about 50 percent carbohydrate (although breakfasts are often much more carb-dense because of the composition of our customary breakfast foods). If the meal is six hundred calories, three hundred of those would be from carbohydrate. This amount of carbohydrate, broken down into grams, is equal to about seventy-five grams. If we use breakfast as an example, where it's not at all unusual to eat seventy-five grams of carb at a sitting,

Three Large Meals

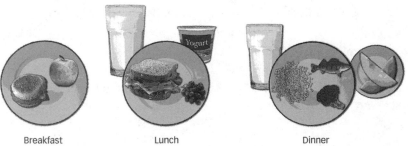

Breakfast   Lunch   Dinner

let's assume your breakfast consists of a deli bagel and a coffee with three teaspoons of sugar, which is approximately seventy-five grams of carb. Once you eat the seventy-five-gram carb breakfast, within an hour the glucose from those carbs is in your blood, and the whole insulin reaction begins. This volume of carbohydrates demands a sizable insulin response.

The Carb-Distributed Diet

Now let's take a look at the second pattern: three smaller meals and two snacks in a day. Assuming the goal is not necessarily to trim calories from the day's meals, the carbohydrate load of this breakfast could be tempered, and redistributed, to command less of an insulin response.

Most bagels are too big, too calorie dense, and too refined to be the best breakfast choice for most people on a regular basis, unless they're exceptionally active (especially when you slather on the typical two tablespoons of cream cheese at fifty calories per tablespoon!). Try changing that sixty-gram carb bagel (roughly four ounces, or 320 calories) to a 100 percent whole grain English muffin, for about thirty grams of carbs; add one tablespoon of peanut butter (negligible carbs); change the sugar to an artificial sweetener (zero carbs), and add an eight-ounce glass of 1 percent milk (twelve grams) for a grand total of forty-two grams of much-better-quality carbohydrate. With these adjustments, you also trimmed about 100 calories from breakfast, with this option weighing in at about 330 calories—a vast improvement over the roughly 430 calories from the bagel with cream cheese and the sugar-laden coffee.

This breakfast choice is also packed with positive nutrition. From a blood sugar standpoint, you've tempered your insulin response by trading a seventy-five-gram carb breakfast for a forty-two-gram carb alternative.

Three Smaller Meals and Two Snacks

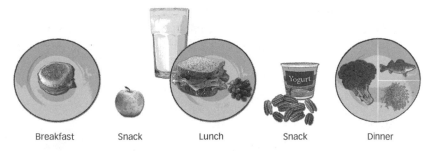

Breakfast   Snack   Lunch   Snack   Dinner

This way, much less insulin will be needed over the next couple of hours to sweep the sugars out of the bloodstream. Once that job is done, there's still room in your carb budget to follow breakfast with a midmorning fruit snack (fifteen grams of carb) two or three hours later.

So there you have it—your first lesson in how to lower your insulin levels. The things you do to lessen your insulin response also often trim calories from your diet without you even focusing on calorie control. There's more than one reason why following a carb-distributed diet may result in weight loss. Beyond the calories saved by trimming carbs, there are several other positive side effects. Transitioning from three larger, more spread-out meals to smaller meals and two snacks helps you to stay ahead of your hunger, which ultimately leads to eating less. Here's why: Human beings are evolutionarily wired to binge eat if we get too hungry. It's actually a leftover caveman survival instinct. In those times it wasn't unusual for people to go fairly long without eating because food was often scarce. But when they did finally kill an antelope, or dig up some edible roots, watch out! They'd eat fast and furious, consuming far more food than they needed that day to stockpile calories for the lean times.

Many of us still do this kind of reactive overeating. We find ourselves in situations where we get busy with our daily activities, forget to eat lunch, and suddenly we notice we're famished sometime in the late afternoon. We then end up eating out of control from dinnertime on. This doesn't happen because you're a weak individual who lacks willpower. After a million-plus years of human evolution, we're conditioned this way! It also could be our brain sensing that blood sugars are drifting too low, signaling that it's time to restock our blood with nutrients.

How do you battle these instincts in modern times? Try to avoid going more than three or four hours without eating a meal or snack. This will help you stay out of the "I'm starving" zone, so you can approach the next meal maybe hungry but not starving. You'll then be in a better position to manage the quality and quantity of your food intake. Another way to look at it is that if you were to rate your hunger on a scale of one to ten (one being "not hungry" and ten being "starved"), you want to eat your next meal or snack when your hunger is a five to six ("somewhat hungry"), instead of waiting for the eight to ten "starved" hunger that will likely lead to overeating.

Avoiding extreme hunger will also help you slow down your eating, which helps control calories. Studies show that the satiety (sense of fullness) signal that travels from your stomach to your brain takes about fifteen or twenty minutes to get there, so eating slowly gives your brain more time to register that you've eaten and that you can stop. Extreme hunger leads to rapid eating that doesn't give your brain a chance to register fullness until after your stomach sends you back to the stove for seconds! You end up cramming loads of calories in, without stopping until you feel stuffed (you know that sensation—the one that says you can't handle even one more bite of that food that tasted so good a minute ago!). This delayed fullness is a major reason why eating too much fast food is such a health hazard. One study found that the average fast food meal takes only about seven minutes to consume, which explains why even a small person can easily consume well over a thousand calories in a short time in these restaurants. Fast food is just that—food that is so effortlessly consumed that your brain doesn't have a prayer of registering that mega-burger and fries until well after the wrappers are in the trash. There's a difference between being "hungry" and "starving," and between being "full" and "stuffed."

Because of the insulin resistance, many women with PCOS are extremely sensitive to blood sugar fluctuations, with significant dips often stimulating sensations of hunger, particularly for carbs. In fact, many of these women describe themselves as carb addicts; they feel like once they start eating carbs, they can't stop! Indulging in carbs does raise the levels of a calming chemical in your brain called serotonin, so it's quite possible that loading up on carbs is a way of self-medicating when we experience stress. But this is really a stress-management issue, which we'll address in chapter 13.

The Carb-Binging Cycle

Many insulin-resistant women describe falling into a cycle that results in reactive binging on carbs. It can start by eating a high-carb meal, particularly one high in processed carbs (for example, a sandwich on white bread and a regular soda or other high-sugar drink). Because insulin-resistant women may overreact with insulin in response to a load of carbohydrate, a couple of hours later this excess circulating insulin may knock their blood sugars down to low levels, making them feel like they have low blood sugar or hypoglycemia. Symptoms of hypoglycemia include hunger, nervousness, perspiration, shakiness, dizziness, light-headedness, sleepiness, and feeling anxious or weak.

This is not the same potentially dangerous state of hypoglycemia that an insulin-dependent diabetic may experience if he or she takes too much insulin. However, if your brain senses your blood sugar levels are dropping below ideal, it's going to start screaming for food (mainly carbs) to replenish blood sugars to a more comfortable level. Many women unknowingly respond to these impulses in the worst possible way—by once again flooding their system with another load of carb, maybe this time in the form of a candy bar from the vending machine at work at four in the afternoon. The most symptomatic patient I ever counseled reacted to a feeling of low blood sugar by downing a large bag of chips and a Mountain Dew! The cycle then repeats itself, although by this time you may be home, overeating at dinner in response to the next round of low blood sugar sensations! Avoiding this cycle comes back to one of the main premises of the carb-distributed diet plan: spreading good-quality carbs out over the day will temper your insulin response and help you avoid wide blood sugar fluctuations that can lead to poor food choices and binge eating.

The carb-distributed diet also helps with weight loss because of how fast and how long you feel full. One of the plan's foundations is to opt for unrefined carbs as much as possible, which means you'll be eating a lot more fiber. Fiber is one of the most fulfilling things you can eat! Fiber is the part of a plant food (from fruits, vegetables, nuts, seeds, beans, and whole grains) that human beings can't digest. Cows can digest fiber, because they are ruminants and have four stomachs for digesting tough food. But for humans, once the digestion process is complete, fiber remains in the intestines, passes through to the colon, and is ultimately eliminated in stool.

How does this help manage insulin resistance and possibly help you lose weight? If some of the carbohydrate you eat is in the form of fiber, some of it will never even make it into your bloodstream, thereby dampening your insulin response. Also, when digestible carbs become intertwined with fiber, your digestive processes are going to have to contend with the fiber to get at the digestible sugars and other nutrients, resulting in a more gradual—and more lasting—release of glucose into the blood. The more gradual the release of sugars into the blood, the longer it will be before you feel hungry again. In your stomach, fiber absorbs water and expands, increasing the sense of fullness these naturally low-calorie foods provide.

Fiber and Weight Control

Many studies correlate high-fiber intake with lasting weight loss, which mainly has to do with how high-fiber foods affect calorie balance. In general, people won't stop eating until they feel physically full. According to researcher Barbara Rolls from Penn State University, part of what leads us to feel full is that we sense a certain volume or density of food in our stomach.[7] If you intentionally eat more plant foods, your stomach will still register food volume, but you'll be filling up on lower-calorie foods that will help to displace higher-calorie foods in your stomach, leading to a satisfying sensation of fullness on fewer calories. Foods that are high in fiber are among the most universally nourishing, with many studies correlating diets high in fiber with lower risks of diabetes, high blood pressure, heart disease, cancer, and other diseases. Not a veggie eater, you say? We'll deal with you later in the book (see chapter 10)!

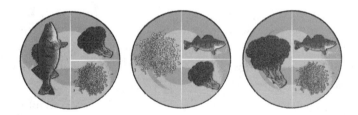

If you look at these three different dinner plates, the first two are most typical of what our dinner plates look like—half the plate is either a large portion of meat or a big pile of starch (like rice, potato, or pasta). The third plate is just as full of food, but half the plate is covered with vegetables. It could be a large serving of cooked vegetables, a salad, or a portion of both. Or it could include some fresh fruit (although that's often eaten after a meal).The idea is that you're still eating a decent-sized plate of food, but it's much lower in calories—and healthier for you—than the first two plates. Countless studies tie higher intake of fruits and vegetables to better success with weight loss, and their function is quite simple: fill your plate up with something healthy, so you'll leave less room on it (and in

> ### *Overcoming Your Animal Instincts*
>
> We have animal instincts in us, but we're the only species of a high enough intelligence to ignore them. Can you imagine trying to talk a lion out of killing an antelope that was right in front of it? Of course not! But you can become a mindful eater by starting to pay attention. Start planning your next meal or snack when your hunger is tapping you on the shoulder instead of waiting for it to slap you in the face! Another advantage of the carb-distributed diet emphasizes the issue of appetite control. Eating smaller amounts of less-refined carbs, particularly when they are paired with protein and a little healthy fat, holds blood sugars steady, which helps you to avoid blood sugar dips that can result in carb cravings.

your stomach) for foods like extra-large portions of meat, chicken or fish, pasta, rice, potatoes, cream or cheese sauces, gravies, and other calorie-dense foods and add-ons that can crank up your calorie intake.

Physical Activity, Dietary Fat, and Medications

In addition to the carb-distributed diet, there are other extremely important players in managing your PCOS that play synergistic roles in helping to get your health and hormones in line. The first major player is exercise, which is so important we've devoted a whole chapter to it (see chapter 7). Exercise is absolutely mandatory for weight loss (particularly for the *maintenance* of weight loss, which is often trickier to master than losing the weight!). It also stimulates the release of chemicals inside cells that enhance the movement of glucose out of the bloodstream and into the cell. This response is so powerful—and so totally natural—that it's the main reason why diabetes was so rare up until recent generations. Plain and simple, throughout most of human history, life was so physically grueling that the struggle was, if anything, to keep weight on. Up until the past two or three generations, life was hard work! People worked on farms or in factories for long hours, doing intense physical work that burned hundreds if not thousands of calories a day. Food was something you had to hunt and gather, then you had to skin it, clean it, and build a fire to cook it—all of which burned a lot of calories.

Although much of this is still true for people living in developing countries, in the United States, and increasingly in many other industrialized countries, these intense activities of daily living are almost nonexistent.

We don't chop wood or shovel coal to heat our houses. We may have a garden, but we're certainly not out logging miles through the woods gathering nuts, seeds, grasses, and berries, never mind hunting down animals for our dinner. And unless you're loading boxes for UPS, doing the heavy lifting at a construction site, or working alongside your clients as a personal trainer, the chances you're burning many calories on the job—or kicking up high levels of these glucose-clearing enzymes in your cells—is slim to none. I certainly don't do it much on my job. I'm either sitting at my desk writing or sitting in an office counseling patients. Life as it exists today for many of us is very conducive to developing "diabesity"—the far-too-common pairing of diabetes and obesity that is exploding in the U.S. population. But, rest assured, you don't have to go back to living on the prairie! Even small amounts of exercise consistently added to your day can yield vast improvements in your health.

Another major player in dealing with your PCOS is fat. The type and amount of fat you eat is important for managing both your weight and your insulin resistance. Studies show that saturated fats may worsen insulin resistance, and it's suspected that trans fats may do the same. Whether substituting heart-healthy unsaturated fats for saturated and trans fats can improve insulin resistance is still being studied, but it could be that lowering your risk of heart disease may trickle down to managing insulin resistance. This could be more evidence that feeding your body the way it's genetically designed to be fed improves health in many ways. Many diseases affect each other. For example, being overweight increases your risk of diabetes and dementia, so what's good for your weight is good for your heart and your brain as well. Obesity and insulin resistance are also risk factors for cancer, which many people are not aware of.

The final player in managing your PCOS might be medications. My goal is to help you manage your health and hormones as naturally as possible through diet and lifestyle change (activity, sensible supplementation, stress management, and so on). But despite your best efforts, sometimes medications are needed to help regulate your menstrual cycles, control your symptoms, manage your health risk factors, or help you see your way clear to what needs to happen to get better. Some problems you may be experiencing, like hypothyroidism, don't respond to diet or exercise. In other situations it could be that what's happening with your health has been going on for a while and has progressed to the point where you need to start medications now to get better. For example, maybe you're already showing signs of prediabetes and medications may help you reduce your risk of progressing to full-blown diabetes.

There's also the possibility of starting out on medications that you can wean off of down the road as the effects of diet and lifestyle change take hold. Or you may only need medications temporarily to increase your odds of getting pregnant. The point is to be open to medication if it makes sense in your situation. There's an awful lot we can do to keep our dependence on medications to a minimum, however. If you want to find out whether medications may be appropriate for you, have that discussion with a clinician experienced in managing women with PCOS. Be sure you understand why you're taking what's prescribed.

. . .

The steps you take to manage your PCOS—through diet and lifestyle change, and possibly with assistance from medications if appropriate—can positively influence your health in many ways. Gaining control of your PCOS symptoms will help you feel more energetic, less emotionally volatile, less stressed-out, and more optimistic that you can take charge of your health.

PART 2

Managing Health and Hormones through Diet and Lifestyle

4

The Carbohydrate-
Distributed Diet

Now that you have a better understanding of how diet and exercise can help you manage your PCOS, let's talk specifics. How do you make this happen? It's important to be able to short-circuit any negative thinking that may sabotage your ability to make change. Sometimes, simply understanding why we do some of the crazy things we do when it comes to food can be very helpful. It's tough but entirely possible to rewire your thought processes toward more positive thinking.

Women with PCOS are at high risk for jumping on the low-carb bandwagon, given the connection between carbs and insulin needs. The problem with this approach is that it completely ignores the legions of research supporting the value of including good-quality carbs in the diet for prevention of such diseases as heart disease, diabetes, and cancer. Low-carb diets have also not been proven to result in lasting weight loss. Having said that, there is always room for improvement in the way most women with PCOS—or average Americans, for that matter—consume carbohydrates.

Consider these facts: Most Americans eat too many calories. According to the Centers for Disease Control, Americans are consuming more calories than they did thirty years ago, and the rate of increase is three times greater in women than men. U.S. women increased their daily calorie consumption 22 percent between 1971 and 2000, from 1,542 calories per day to 1,877 calories. During the same period the calorie intake for men increased 7 percent, from 2,450 calories per day to 2,618 calories. Most of the calorie increase during that period came from increasing our intake of carbohydrates. Men increased the percentage of their daily calorie intake from carbohydrates from 42.4 to 49 percent. Women increased their carbohydrate consumption from 45.4 to 51.6 percent of daily calorie intake.

When it comes to the kinds of carbohydrates we eat, Americans tend to have a preference for sugar and refined, or white flour, carbohydrates. These findings are from the most recent National Health and Nutrition Examination Survey (NHANES) conducted by the CDC's National Center for Health Statistics in 1999–2000, which describes trends in our daily food intake over the past three decades.[1] The last food trends survey occurred before the low-carb bubble and bust, so it's possible that some shifts have happened in Americans' eating habits since then. But the fact remains that we have gotten heavier than ever over the past two decades—the result of too many calories from all types of sources and not enough physical activity.

The Land of Carb Addicts

Many readers may be too young to remember the "fat-free" 1980s. At that time a surge of research emerged tying high-fat diets to an increased risk of cardiovascular disease. American diets were becoming increasingly high in fat—as was the average American body—and scientists and health advocates began clamoring for Americans to lower their fat intake to reduce their risk of heart attack and stroke. Their recommendations made sense: fatty foods are high in calories, and every gram of fat we eat deposits nine calories into our system, whereas proteins and carbohydrates deliver only four calories per gram. This country's dieting history is rife with extreme plans: lists of "only eat this" and "never eat that" foods. Many concluded that if less fat is good for you, *no* fat must be better.

I started my professional life as a nutritionist during this time, which I refer to as the "Snackwell era," where fat-free Snackwell cookies and thousands of other fat-free foods flooded the market. Taste began to disappear from food as our focus turned to foods that didn't contain deadly fat. For most people, the replacement food became fat-free carbs. Unless they're fried or drowned in cheese, butter, or creamy sauces, most carbohydrates are naturally low or devoid of fat. For the first time, four- to five-ounce gigantic bagels came out of the Jewish delis and into the mainstream. Rice and pasta reigned supreme, and everyone's favorite treat eventually became available in a low-fat or fat-free version.

Anyone who lived through that fad will tell you that many of the market's responses to the fat-free craze fell flat: fat-free cheese was foul, foods didn't brown in the oven, and that intangible quality that we call "mouthfeel" went out the window. But Americans did learn to eat less fat. Unfortunately, we also continued to get fatter. After a few years on the fat-free bandwagon, it started to become clear that a fat-free diet may take a bite out of our blood cholesterol (studies show a decline in blood cholesterol levels from the early 1980s to 2002; in part this was also a result of increased use of cholesterol-lowering medications at this time), but it was not going to be the solution to our ever-expanding waistlines. There are actually several problems with the fat-free approach:

- Most carbs contain little to no protein, which we now realize helps provide a feeling of fullness for a longer period of time after a meal.
- Most people were opting for refined, processed carbohydrates that had been stripped of their fiber—another nutrient we now know helps us feel fuller for longer after a meal.
- Many people adopted a subconscious attitude that if something was "fat free," you could eat as much as you wanted. But carbohydrates still contain calories! If you nibbled on them all day long—which many people did because refined carbs don't control hunger for very long—you could still up end up consuming more calories than you need.
- Some fat also makes food taste good and helps us to feel full.

The overriding lesson of the fat-free trend was that weight loss and health didn't result from taking all the fat out of your diet. Some fats are actually good for you, like the healthful fats found in fish and monounsaturated fats (like olive and canola oil, nuts, seeds, and avocado) and the polyunsaturated fats in seeds and vegetable oils. These fats may actually reduce your risk of cardiovascular disease and enhance the absorption of healthful fat-soluble vitamins (like A, D, E, and K) and phytonutrients (such as the health-promoting lycopene in tomatoes). Fat holds our hunger at bay longer than fat-free foods. And a little bit of fat makes people happy! Its rich taste and creamy mouthfeel enhances the enjoyment of many of the foods we love.

The bottom line on fat comes down to the principle of the Two Qs— quality and quantity. Some fat is good for you if you choose the right type and watch how much you eat. Many of us could have saved ourselves from another fad if instead of turning away from too much fat and toward refined carbohydrates, we opted for whole grains. But we didn't. We needed to learn the Two Qs lesson about carbohydrates from the low-carb frenzy that would follow about a decade later. As Americans, we try every new fad, thinking the "right" diet is high in one thing and low in something else. But for women with PCOS and other forms of insulin resistance, your best bet is a less-processed, moderate carbohydrate diet, where carbs are spread out in smaller doses over meals and snacks, paired with lean proteins and small amounts of healthful fats wherever possible.

Carbohydrates: The Basics

As a source of easy-to-access energy, carbohydrates are critical to everyone's diet. Carbs can be quickly converted to glucose, which acts as a fuel source for every cell in the body. The key is to choose the best-quality carbohydrates and watch the quantity you consume (the Two Qs mentioned earlier). Even the most recent U.S. Dietary Guidelines on the percentage of calories that should come from carbohydrate, proteins, and fats acknowledge that the best diet for an individual is not one-size-fits-all. What too often gets lost in the discussion about carbohydrates is the incredibly valuable role they play in keeping us healthy and feeling energetic—if you choose the right ones. Foods that contain carbohydrates make many valuable contributions to the human body. Carbs are the body's main source of fuel as they are easily broken down into glucose, the "gasoline" of the human body.

Although glucose is used as a fuel source for every cell in the body, the biggest consumers of glucose are muscles and the central nervous system (the brain, spinal cord, and nerves). In fact, brain cells need twice as much energy as the other cells in the body. The central nervous system needs about four hundred to six hundred calories' worth of carbohydrate a day for those tissues to be fully fueled, accounting for the sensations of weakness and moodiness, trouble focusing, and in some people actual shakiness, when we go too long without eating. In many people these symptoms cause intense cravings for—you guessed it—carbohydrates!

This explains why some people simply could not tolerate the protein and fat-heavy Atkins diet (officially called the Atkins Nutritional Approach) or the basically carb-free two-week induction phase of the popular South Beach diet. These plans physically made them sick!

Carbohydrates are classified as either complex carbohydrates (also referred to as starches) or sugars. Starches are long chains of sugar units all hooked together. Because starches are large molecules, when they hit your tongue they can't burrow into your taste buds to impart the taste of sweetness. But during digestion, the sugar units are all separated from one another by digestive enzymes and are ultimately released into the bloodstream in their most basic form, as simple sugars (glucose, galactose, and fructose), with glucose being the main form used for energy. Your best choices for complex carbohydrates (starches) are minimally refined whole grains that have retained their dietary fiber and health-promoting phytonutrients because they have not been processed to remove the fiber and the germ (where most of the nutrients are). Refined carbohydrates—like white rice, regular pasta, processed cereals, and other grains made with white flour—have been stripped of their fiber and phytonutrients. Although in the United States most refined carbs are fortified with some vitamins, iron, and other minerals, you can't add back the phytonutrients. They're gone forever.

Unlike starches, which are long chains of sugar units, sugars are either single-unit molecules (glucose, fructose, and galactose) that can be absorbed whole or two units hooked together (sucrose, lactose, and maltose) that need to break down into single units for absorption. Some people lack enough of the enzyme lactase that breaks lactose down into glucose and galactose, causing symptoms of lactose intolerance (with the accompanying symptoms of diarrhea, bloating, and gas). Sugars are small molecules so they can get right into your taste buds and stimulate the sensation of "sweet." Sugars can be either naturally occurring in fruit and dairy foods (packaged along with other healthful nutrients) or added during processing (straight calories with no healthful nutrients).

Most vegetables contain very little carbohydrate. They're made mostly of water and some fiber. For this reason they make a great filler food, and we don't officially count them as carbohydrate foods in discussions about managing carbohydrate intake. There is, however, a short list of starchy vegetables that we count as starch choices at a meal. These include potatoes, sweet potatoes, yams, winter squash, corn, peas, beans, and plantains. You want to consider starchy vegetables as starch when meal planning. Don't eliminate them from the diet; just count them toward the starchy part of the meal. French fries—sadly listed as the number-one consumed vegetable in the United States—should not be regularly counted as a starch. Rather, these should be placed on the "occasional treat list" as they are often fried in unhealthy saturated and trans fats.

Choosing moderate amounts of whole grains, starchy vegetables, and beans to provide the bulk of your carbohydrate intake will add a lot of fiber and other health-promoting nutrients to your diet. Mistakenly focusing on all carbohydrates as "bad for you" and cutting them out of your diet will likely leave you feeling deprived and rob you of many nutrients your body needs for good health and optimal function. It's all about the quality and the quantity! The 2005 U.S. Dietary Guidelines for Americans made many recommendations regarding carbs.[2] The Recommended Dietary Allowance (RDA) for carbohydrates, which should be viewed as the bare minimum for good health and energy, is 130 grams, far more than was allowed on the popular Atkins diet. What exactly does 130 grams of carbohydrates look like? Four servings of grains, two servings of fruits, two servings of dairy (milk or yogurt), and three servings of nonstarchy vegetables.

Sugars can be naturally present in foods (such as the fructose in fruit or the lactose in milk) or sugars can be added to foods, like sugars or syrups that are added at the table or during processing or preparation. One of the most ubiquitous forms of added sugar in today's typical American

The Skinny on Artificial Sweeteners

As concern about excessive intake of carbohydrates has increased, an ever-expanding list of artificial sweeteners has appeared in the food supply. Those currently available include aspartame (NutraSweet, Equal), saccharin (Sweet'N Low, Sugar Twin), sucralose (Splenda), asulfamine K (Sweet One, Sunett), and stevia (Truvia, PureVia). Artificial sweeteners are regulated by the Food and Drug Administration and are generally recognized as safe. With the exception of light yogurt, my feeling is that artificially sweetened foods and beverages are generally highly processed foods devoid of healthful nutrients, so they should ideally be limited to a serving or two a day.

The Glycemic Index

During the low-carb diet days people started to become familiar with the term GI, or glycemic index. The glycemic index is a numerical system that rates how fast carbs from food arrive in your blood as glucose in the hours after you eat. The original research was conducted more than 20 years ago and was designed to help people with diabetes determine how different foods might affect their blood sugar. To determine GI, a 50-gram portion of a carbohydrate-containing food is fed to nondiabetic volunteers, and their blood glucose levels are checked at intervals over the following hours. The standard that foods are compared to is a 50-gram dose (3 tablespoons) of pure oral glucose, which has a rating of 100. The test food is rated based on the percent it raises blood sugar compared to oral glucose (for example, brown rice raises blood sugar 55 percent as much as glucose, so the GI is 55).

Several factors affect GI, including acidity, how much a food is processed or cooked, if it contains fiber, and whether it is eaten with another food. Basically, anything that speeds up a food's digestion will raise its GI. Portion also limits how much any food can raise blood sugar levels regardless of GI. Some foods—like big bagels—can easily deliver a 50-gram dose of carbs, whereas other foods—like carrots, for example, which were routinely bashed for having a high GI—are rarely eaten in 50-gram doses (that's about $1^1/_2$ pounds of carrots!) or alone without other foods present. As you can see, strictly avoiding certain foods with a high GI can deprive you of some very healthful foods.

Another system has been developed called glycemic load that takes into account the GI and the amount of carbohydrates in a serving (within which carrots rate very favorably). A low GL is less than 10, moderate is 11 to 19, and high is 20 or above. The simple interpretation of this is that the more processed and lower in fiber a carbohydrate is, the faster it will break down into glucose, and the more carbs in a portion the higher the blood sugar will eventually rise.[3]

Choosing carbs according to the Two Qs encourages higher-quality carbs and reinforces watching the quantity. Pairing carbohydrates with proteins and healthy fats as we do in the PCOS diet plan will also temper the effect on blood sugar of any carbohydrate. The GI can be a useful system, as long as the quantity issue is also accounted for—just because a food has a low GI does not mean you can eat all you want—and you don't use it as a reason to avoid foods you intuitively know are healthful. For more on the GI and GL of foods visit www.glycemicindex.com.

diet is high-fructose corn syrup, used in sweetened beverages and baked products. The "sugar" content listed on a food label includes both naturally occurring and added sugars. To see how much of this sugar is likely to be added, look at the ingredient label. The closer to the top a sugar is listed, the higher the content of added sugars. In contrast, even though all the carbohydrate in 100 percent orange juice is naturally occurring fructose from the oranges, on the food label it looks like OJ is loaded with "sugar," but the ingredient list shows only oranges and maybe water, no added sugars.

Any of the following terms indicate an added sugar:

Brown sugar	Invert sugar
Corn sweetener	Lactose
Corn syrup	Maltose
Dextrose	Malt syrup
Fructose	Molasses
Fruit juice concentrates	Raw sugar
Glucose	Sucrose
High-fructose corn syrup	Sugar
Honey	Syrup

The body's response to sugars is basically the same (with some fluctuation in insulin response based on glycemic index), whether the sugars are naturally present or added to the food. Natural sugars from fruit (fructose) and dairy (lactose) have an advantage because they're packaged along with other healthful nutrients. Added sugars supply calories but few or no nutrients. Eating a lot of added sugars has been tied to weight gain and poor-quality diets. The majority of our fruit servings should come from whole fruit. One serving a day of 100 percent fruit juice can add some important vitamins and minerals to the diet, but drinking too much can contribute to unwanted weight gain. A serving of juice is one cup according to the Food Pyramid, but only half a cup according to the Exchange Lists for Diabetes (see page 92). Dried fruit can be included as well, but only about two tablespoons will give you the same carb and calorie load as a whole piece of fruit. Legumes—such as dry beans and peas—are especially rich in fiber and protein and should be consumed several times per week.

At least three of your grain servings (or half or more of all your grains) should come from whole grains. Try whole grain cereal, bread, and crackers, brown rice, and whole wheat pasta. Nutrient-rich whole grains have been linked to lower rates of obesity, heart disease, and diabetes, and are more filling than refined carbohydrates. The percentage of calories that should come from carbohydrates ranges from 45 percent to 65 percent depending on health needs (lower in the case of insulin resistance, higher for endurance athletes). Because refined sugar adds so little value to the diet, intake should be limited. Dietary fiber intake should be fourteen grams per every thousand calories consumed, or on average between twenty and thirty-five grams of fiber a day. Dietary surveys suggest we only eat about half that, or fourteen grams a day. Ideally, we would get the bulk of that fiber from naturally occurring fibers in whole grains, fruits, and vegetables as opposed to foods that have fibers added to them (like yogurt or white bread with added fibers). Some of these foods can be included in reasonable amounts but won't count as one of your three whole grain servings.

There is ample reason to include some good-quality carbs in your diet. Quality carbs provide fiber, phytonutrients (health-promoting plant chemicals), and pleasure without loading you down with excess calories. But I'll say it again: it's all about the quantity. There are no free rides when it comes to carbohydrates or any other calorie-containing food for that matter. You can still gain weight on bran cereal, brown rice, or whole wheat pasta if you eat more than you need to balance your calorie intake and activity.

Crunching the Numbers: Calculating Calories and Carbs

An individualized approach is needed to determine how much carbohydrate you should eat to meet your needs without overrestricting the carbs that will do your body good. The best way to do this is to start by estimating your calorie needs and then figure out how much of that should come from carbohydrate, assuming that with insulin resistance aiming for around 45 percent of your calories from carbohydrate is the right amount (some may choose to go lower, but I wouldn't dip below 40 percent). There are several simple ways to estimate your calories, the most user-friendly being those available on the Internet. Many online calorie estimators will ask for various combinations of your age, weight, height, sex, and activity level, then estimate your calorie needs for maintenance of your current weight. You adjust that number based on whether you want to maintain, lose, or gain weight.

One such tool is available on the USDA's MyPyramid.gov website. Enter your data (age, sex, height, weight, and activity level) into the MyPyramid Plan interactive tool and an estimate of how many calories you should aim for will pop up (along with some kindly worded feedback on whether it might be good for you to aim for less!). If you prefer the old-fashioned long-hand way of crunching out your calories, you can also use the Harris Benedict Equation, used by nutrition professionals since 1919 to calculate calorie needs.[4] You will definitely need a calculator. Here's how it works:

- First, calculate your basal metabolic rate (BMR), which tells you how many calories you burn at rest just keeping yourself alive (basically the caloric cost of breathing, keeping your heart beating, digesting food, maintaining your muscles and other organs, and so on). For women this is the formula (using pounds and inches—the original equation uses kilograms and centimeters): 665 + (4.35 × weight in pounds) + (4.7 × height in inches) − (4.7 × age). For men: 066 + (6.23 × weight in pounds) ι (12.7 × height in inches) − (6.8 × age).

- Once you've calculated your BMR, you then need to multiply that number by an "activity factor" that adds on additional calories needed for activity: light activity up to three times a week = BMR × 1.375; moderate activity three to five times a week = BMR × 1.55; vigorous activity six to seven times per week = BMR × 1.725; and extreme activity/intense sports training six to seven days per week = BMR × 1.9.

Let's run through an example using a thirty-five-year-old woman who weighs 185 pounds and is five feet seven inches tall: 665 + 805 (185 pounds × 4.35) + 315 (67 inches × 4.7) − 165 (35 years × 4.7) = 1620 calories for BMR. Her current activity is light, so we take her BMR of 1,620 calories × 1.375 = 2,228 calories. Remember, this number is to *maintain* her weight, so for weight loss she'd need to routinely eat less and exercise more to reach a calorie deficit. When you run these numbers through the MyPyramid Plan on the USDA's website, you get almost the exact same number (2,200 calories) for maintenance.

In this example MyPyramid Plan points out that this weight is higher than desired for good health and offers meal plans for both maintenance at this weight and an alternative 1,800-calorie plan "to gradually move toward a healthier weight." This is an important point, because the calorie-crunching strategies just outlined are to *maintain* your weight. To *lose* weight, the conventional wisdom is that if you want to aim for about one pound of weight loss per week, you should trim 500 calories from your diet. This is based on the assumption that a pound of body fat is equal to about 3,500 calories, so eating 500 calories less for seven days theoretically should result in a one-pound loss of body fat. For many of us, however, cutting 500 calories is too extreme—our brain will definitely notice their absence, possibly ramping up our preoccupation with food. A better alternative—and one that recognizes the mandatory contribution of regular physical activity to weight loss—is to trim about 200 to 300 calories a day from your diet and add in an equal amount of calories burned through physical activity.

If you're really stressed about cutting calories and want to take things slower, cut even fewer calories and get serious with the exercise, aiming for as close to an hour as possible at least five days a week. You'll likely still lose some weight but eventually hit a plateau where you aren't losing anymore, at which point you may be ready to lower your calorie intake further. Research suggests that you can trim your food intake by about 20 percent and still fly below the radar of that monitoring system in your brain that is constantly on the lookout for signs that the food supply might be drying up.[5] Again, better to go slow and steady, focusing on making permanent changes that can stick, rather than repeating a pattern you likely experienced before—cutting a lot of calories and losing weight fast, only to regain it "with interest" when your ability to tolerate the drastic change burns out.

No calorie calculator can take into account body composition—there will always be people who weigh more because they have more lean muscle, which only very expensive, high-tech body composition analysis machines can figure out. Once you have you crunched out your calories, to figure out the calories that should come from carbohydrates, and then the grams, take your total calorie number and multiply it by 0.45 (because we're aiming for 45 percent of calories from carbs). That is a rough estimate of the number of calories you should eat from carbohydrates in a day. For example, let's say your estimated needs are 2,000 calories a day. Take $2,000 \times 0.45 = 900$ carb calories. However, food labels don't list carb calories—they list grams. There are 4 calories per gram of carbohydrate, so if you take that 900 and divide it by 4, you'll get your total grams of carbohydrate for the day, which in this example would be 225 grams of carbohydrate a day. This amount of carbohydrate would be divided over three meals and (ideally) at least one or two snacks.

Food labels that list the Recommended Daily Values from total fat, saturated fat, cholesterol, sodium, total carbohydrates, and dietary fiber are based on a 2,000-calorie diet. This is referred to as the "Footnote" of the Nutrition Facts Label and looks like this:

		Calories: 2,000	2,500
Total Fat	Less than	65g	80g
Sat Fat	Less than	20g	25g
Cholesterol	Less than	300mg	300mg
Sodium	Less than	2,400mg	2,400mg
Total Carbohydrate		300g	375g
Dietary Fiber		25g	30g

*Percent Daily Values are based on a 2,000 calorie diet. Your Daily Values may be higher or lower depending on your calorie needs:

The Recommended Daily Value for carbohydrate based on a 2,000-calorie diet is 300 grams a day. Our calculation for someone with insulin resistance recommends about 225 grams of carb per day, which would be your "allowance" of carbohydrates to work with over the day. This is 25 percent below the usual recommendation for carbohydrate, but notice that I am not recommending a "low-carb" diet. Compare this to the 25 grams of carb a day that are recommended during the induction phase of the Atkins diet. Limiting your carbs that severely may have helped you lose weight in the short run if you could tolerate it, but some people got monster headaches and developed serious irritability problems when they subjected their brain and nervous system to so little carbohydrate. In the long term it's neither healthy nor realistic to stick to consuming so little carbohydrate.

Distributing Your Carb Budget throughout the Day

Once you have your carbohydrate budget figured out, you need to determine how to best distribute them throughout the day. If you come up with 225 grams of carb, it's not going to help if you decide to divide them into two huge meals that are roughly 112 grams each. Eating this large a load of carbohydrate at one sitting is likely to result in a pretty large bolus of glucose release into your blood an hour later, with a subsequent hefty release of insulin into your system. Assuming a healthier eating pattern of three meals a day, a much more reasonable amount of carbohydrate to consume at one meal is in the 45- to 60-gram range. When it comes to eating, aiming for a range is a good thing. It prevents you from obsessing about a specific number and allows for some flexibility. Given that carbohydrates yield 4 calories per gram, 45 grams of carbohydrate is 180 calories and 60 grams is 240 calories. Whether you should aim for 45 grams or more like 60 grams of carb largely depends on how much you're trying to control your calories and how hungry you are at the moment. Be sure to keep in mind that the calories from the protein and fat you're eating count toward the total for your meal as well.

Someone with diabetes can see immediate biofeedback about carbohydrate consumption from his or her blood glucose monitoring, so he or she can figure out how much carbohydrate should be eaten at a meal based on what the individual postmeal glucose response is. Both the American Diabetes Association and the American Academy of Endocrinologists make recommendations for what blood glucose levels should be two hours after a meal, and suggest that a reading of less than 180 milligrams per deciliter (mg/dl) is good, and less than 140 mg/dl is better. How much carbohydrate someone with diabetes can get away with eating and still hit this goal can vary—maybe 45 grams, maybe 60 grams, or maybe even 75 grams if that person is large, active, or male (because of larger muscle mass). In other words, those with diabetes can actually see what their body thinks of what they just ate. If it was too much carbohydrate, their blood sugar will be too high after a meal. They can then adjust their carbohydrate intake the next time they eat a similar meal—maybe switch to light bread, move the fruit out of the meal and into a snack later on, or eat a smaller portion of dessert.

Let's construct a daily meal plan based on a sample carb budget of 225 grams, beginning with mealtimes:

Daily Meal Plan 1

Breakfast	60 grams
Lunch	60 grams
Dinner	60 grams
Total	**180 grams**

We've used up 180 grams of our 225-gram budget. That leaves 45 grams of carb left to distribute between snacks. Here's one way to do it:

Daily Meal Plan 2

Breakfast	60 grams
Midmorning snack	15 grams
Lunch	60 grams
Afternoon snack	30 grams
Dinner	60 grams
Total	**225 grams**

Another way to spread the carbs out could look like this:

Daily Meal Plan 3

Breakfast	60 grams
Midmorning snack	15 grams
Lunch	60 grams
Afternoon snack	15 grams
Dinner	60 grams
Evening	15 grams
Total	**225 grams**

How might this be different if you were aiming for a lower calorie intake, such as 1,600 calories? Let's crunch the numbers: $1600 \times 0.45 = 720$ carbohydrate calories. Divide 720 by 4 calories per gram for carbohydrates = 180 grams total carbs for the day. With this lower calorie goal, assume 45 grams of carbohydrate per meal:

Daily Meal Plan 4

Breakfast	45 grams
Lunch	45 grams
Dinner	45 grams
Total	**135 grams**

This leaves us with 45 grams of carbs to spread between snacks, as seen in the fifth meal plan.

Daily Meal Plan 5

Breakfast	45 grams
Midmorning Snack	15 grams
Lunch	45 grams
Afternoon Snack	30 grams*
Dinner	45 grams
Total	**180 grams**

*Note: A 1,400-calorie meal plan would look similar, only the afternoon snack would be 15 grams of carbohydrate instead of 30 grams.

Of course, we haven't factored in the protein and fat calories in these meal plans yet, and all calories count when it comes to losing weight. Once you start being mindful of eating according to a regular meal pattern, prioritizing eating your next meal or snack when you're hungry but not starving, along with quelling your insulin response by curbing the amount of carbohydrates you eat at a meal or snack, it will be easier not to eat too much food. You just won't crave it as much.

Why Distribute the Carbohydrates?

When you eat carbohydrates, within an hour the majority of that carbohydrate has been digested and released as glucose into the blood. The goal of the carb-distributed plan is to maintain a sustained blood glucose level that fluxes within a steady range—not too high, not too low—so your blood glucose levels are rolling like hills, not widely varying in a mountains-and-valleys pattern. When you eat a moderate amount of carbohydrate at once, you get a more muted insulin release that should help bring glucose levels back to baseline without overshooting the mark (and causing sensations of low blood sugar and subsequent hunger). With a large load of carbohydrate eaten at once, you'll likely respond with a more aggressive insulin release, which can lower your blood glucose levels—sometimes too much—causing an abrupt decline in glucose levels that deprives your central nervous system and muscles of a steady fuel source. This triggers hunger as a means of repleting blood glucose levels to a steady state.

If you eat a breakfast of forty-five to sixty grams of carbohydrate, depending on how hungry you tend to get, a few hours later it may make sense to have a snack of fruit or some other small portion of carbohydrate (with or without a small amount of protein) to keep yourself from becoming too hungry by lunchtime. Lunch and dinner are usually significantly farther apart, so a planned protein-plus-carb snack eaten midafternoon, when you're maybe a little hungry but not starving, can go a long way toward preventing extreme hunger and overeating. If you don't want to overeat, eat frequently enough to help keep your hunger in check. According to the National Weight Control Registry, successful weight losers eat four to five times a day (see chapter 6 for more on this idea).

Defining a Carbohydrate

The short answer is that anything that comes from a plant contains carbohydrates. Fruits, vegetables (although starchy vegetables are the only significant sources), and grains all contain carbohydrates. Milk and yogurt also contain carbohydrate in the form of lactose. Although cheese is made from milk, most of the carbohydrate is consumed by the healthy bacteria used to make the cheese, so cheese contains little to no carbohydrate. These "good carbs" contribute a lot of healthy nutrients to the diet in addition to glucose for energy. Then there are the empty-calorie carbs that have little to offer nutritionally beyond glucose calories (soda, candy, cakes, cookies, ice cream, chips, and other snack foods). These foods provide few vitamins and minerals, no fiber, are often vehicles for large amounts of unhealthy trans and saturated fats, and are the source of many excess calories.

Americans consume too much added sugar and nutrient-poor refined carbohydrates, and too few healthful, unprocessed carbohydrates that can do the body good. It's not that there's no room for special treats. Even the USDA's MyPyramid allows for some "discretionary calories" once your other needs for healthful foods are met. If you go out of your way to include fruits and vegetables at meals and snacks, it's possible to make room for a small serving of something to indulge your sweet tooth (or whatever your special treat happens to be). There are several ways to manage the amount of carbohydrate you're eating. Which one you prefer to use largely depends on what kind of approach you'd like to take, and how much you like to control the variables. My personal preference is to start with general changes, knowing you can always control things in a tighter fashion as time goes on and you reassess your needs.

Slower weight loss is more likely to be permanent because slower loss tends to reflect that you're making slow, cumulative changes over time. You're transitioning from an old set of unhealthful habits to some new ones. Small changes that build on each other over time are generally more successful at permanently changing your diet and lifestyle routines—the habits you default to every day when the alarm goes off and your feet hit the floor. Our weight and health is where it is in part because of our genes but also because of the patterns we've established over time, maybe since childhood. Those patterns need to change, and they need to change permanently, to prevent you from drifting back to old routines. But you don't have to be perfect! Remember that 80/20 rule: it's your habits that affect your weight and health, not the occasional special indulgence.

The bottom line is that diet, lifestyle, and weight change take time and hard work. Changing lifestyle habits is a bit like getting a new job. Many people stay in jobs they hate or that they know are leading nowhere, because at least they know what to expect when they walk through the door in the morning. Finding a new job requires work: researching what's out there, taking inventory of your skills, making sure you're prepared with the right outfit or equipment for the new job, and putting on a positive face for the potential new employer. You reach a point of readiness to look for a new job and eventually land one.

How do you feel when you first get a new job? Excited, optimistic that you're making a good choice. But there's also usually some apprehension— you don't know the responsibilities yet, or the people, or exactly where you fit in. You may need to follow someone around, keep lots of lists, and focus on every detail in the beginning. In a reasonably short time, though, you're walking through the door and jumping into the job with relative ease. Why? Because you're repeating the new skills you're being trained in every day. If you want to keep the job, honing those skills isn't optional! Unfortunately, we don't allocate the same due diligence to lifestyle change. Whether we have food in the house, whether we push back on everything else in our busy lives (including the job) to make sure we make time to eat before we get starved and out of control, and whether we chisel a few minutes out of each day to move our body in a way that preserves our muscles, burns calories, and short-circuits stress will make all the difference. I know, it's not easy. But nothing we do that's monumental in our lives, that really has the ability to change our circumstances in a positive way, is easy. One of the most beautiful things about eating better and exercising regularly is that it tends to change us both inside and out, which trickles down to many other things that affect our quality of life in a positive way.

Three Steps to Making Dietary Change

In the extremely insightful words of my professional mentor and friend Dr. Margo Woods, a nutrition professor and researcher at the world-renowned Tufts University School of Nutrition in Boston, "Dietary change is a three-step process that people need to move through, but often we quit when we're only halfway there!" Those three steps look roughly like this:

Step 1. Start by purging a lot of the refined foods from your diet, those that are filling you up and racking up the calories without adding any nutritional value. There's no need to construct lists of foods you can never eat again, but get real about what should be on your "eat most of the time" list (fruits, vegetables, whole grains, low-fat dairy, and lean protein foods like seafood, poultry, soy foods,

Mind-Set Intervention: Diet and Behavior Change

Changing your eating habits is not necessarily about knowing the facts. I've been a nutrition counselor for more than two decades and worked with many highly educated, even brilliant people who know what to do but struggle to make it happen. The key to making change is to accept that diet and lifestyle change begins in your head and works its way down. You have to be mentally ready to do it and accept that we're not talking about making temporary changes to lose weight. One of the hardest things to do can be to shake free of your past experiences and expectations of weight loss. The most challenging part tends to be how fast you should expect to lose weight.

Dieting in our culture has largely been about making extreme changes abruptly, often using dietary strategies that can't or shouldn't be sustained long term, with a goal of losing weight. The subconscious message is that if we're just good enough, we'll lose the excess weight, pack it up in a trunk, and ship it off to a foreign country from which it will never return. The reality is the weight you lost is just sitting on the sidelines, waiting for you to drift back to the lifestyle habits that didn't serve you well before the diet. Research tells us that weight lost as a result of temporary changes has an extremely slim chance of staying off, largely because "will-powering" yourself to follow a set of food rules for a period of time without doing the hard work of permanently changing the way you approach food and activity has very little likelihood of sticking.

and beans) versus your "eat less often" list (sweets, salty snacks, fatty foods, and fast food).

Step 2. Start to incorporate healthier foods into your diet by over-hauling one meal or one snack at a time. Substitute reduced-fat cheese and crackers for that afternoon vending-machine snack. Replace the snack cake for dessert at lunch with some fruit salad. Switch out the full-fat mayo in the tuna from the office cafeteria with some tuna with reduced-fat mayo from home. If you keep at these one-at-a-time changes, you will eventually arrive at step 3 . . .

Step 3. Consistently eating healthier. This means eating three meals and one or two snacks a day of whole, unrefined foods—whole grain breads, cereals, and crackers, whole fruits, lots of vegetables, low or reduced-fat dairy, and reasonable-sized portions of seafood, poultry, or lean meat, maybe including a vegetarian meal once or twice a week. All this while occasionally incorporating in a small portion of something sweet, or fatty, or whatever your favorite treat is. Keep a realistic eye on how many calories these treats are contrib-uting to your daily diet.

Unfortunately we often run out of steam at step 2 because we get impa-tient, we aren't losing enough weight, or we simply are not used to this gradual approach. But the rewards start kicking in at step 3. You have to leave room for struggles and lapses—hang in there! It's an uphill bat-tle in this obesity-inducing culture, and you have to get used to a little discomfort. But if you've been around the block without lasting success and now your health or fertility are at stake, do you really have a choice? What is there to lose spending the next few months trying to develop some new habits instead of gaining more weight and feeling progressively uncomfortable—and unhappy?

The Balanced-Plate Approach

To increase your odds of success, I recommend starting with small changes and building on them over time. The balanced-plate approach incorpo-rates counting carbohydrates as a means of controlling the amount of carbs you eat. Contrary to the typical American diet, where half the plate is protein (like meat or chicken) or half the plate is starch (rice, potato, or pasta), with this approach half the plate is nonstarchy vegetables. The idea is to play with what's on your plate so you're visually satisfied with the volume of food; you want it to appear that there's enough food there so that you're not being overly deprived. The net effect of what happens in your bloodstream and metabolism after using the balanced-plate approach is conducive to lowering your circulating insulin levels and curbing your calorie intake. Let's break it down into steps.

Balanced Plate: Step 1

 Cover half your plate with nonstarchy vegetables. Let's start with a few assumptions and some important information to help understand this veggie-heavy approach. The size of the plate matters. Studies show that the bigger the plate, the more we tend to eat. In the 1980s plates averaged ten inches in diameter. Today they average twelve inches across. Dinner plates a century ago were the size of modern-day salad plates. Try starting your meal with a salad, then have the rest of your dinner on the same plate. This trick will also save on after-dinner cleanup! The main reason for covering half your plate with vegetables is to help take up space in your stomach with foods that are low in carbohydrates and calories. Part of what contributes to the biological process of feeling full is that your stomach stretches out, triggering the release of chemicals that contribute to that feeling of fullness. If you don't have any vegetables on your plate, by default you'll be relying on more calorie-dense foods—like meat, chicken, cheese, bread, pasta, rice, and potatoes—to do all the stretching. You want less room on your plate and in your stomach for carb and calorie-rich food.

Covering half your plate with vegetables is healthy for loads of reasons. Not only will it help you lose weight and blunt your insulin response, it will also lower your risk of heart disease, cancer, and other chronic health problems. Vegetables can be a combination of cooked and raw. Maybe you have a salad with low-fat dressing before the meal, which may help fill you up and blunt your appetite, then a cooked vegetable with the meal. You could also start a meal with a broth-based vegetable soup (studies show soups also help fill you up on the front end of the meal) to help reduce your intake of the more calorie-dense foods served later in the meal. When choosing vegetables, mix it up to include a variety of colors.

Besides diversifying your intake of vitamins and minerals, many of the health-promoting nutrients in plant foods (phytonutrients) are the same compounds that give a plant its color.

If you historically haven't been a vegetable eater, now is the time to start retrying all those vegetables you assume you don't like to see if your taste has changed. Just because you hated your mother's overcooked string beans when you were a kid (sorry, Mom—a common complaint among my clients!) doesn't mean you'll dislike string beans sautéed in olive oil, garlic, and a little salt and pepper. Taste does change over time, but you'll never know if you don't take a chance and experiment. Try them raw, steamed, sautéed in olive oil and garlic, tossed in lemon juice or balsamic vinegar, mixed into a soup, on top of a pizza, or grilled on the barbeque. Experimenting with vegetables at a friend's house, in a restaurant, or at sampling stations in a produce market are great opportunities to try something new.

Balanced Plate: Step 2

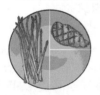

Cover about 25 percent of your plate with lean protein, includ-ing some plant sources. If there's one thing we learned from the low-carb craze, it's that protein is important. Protein lends a feeling of fullness to a meal and keeps you feeling fuller longer. Think about it—how long does a salad with fat-free dressing last you before you feel hungry again? What about if you add some grilled chicken, a hard-boiled egg, or some beans? Adding protein definitely holds hunger at bay. Because the same fats that are bad for your heart (saturated and trans fats) appear to worsen insulin resistance, it's important to pick lean sources of protein, like these:

- Chicken or turkey breast (not fried)
- Fish and seafood (not fried)
- Lean meat (anything with the words "loin," "round," or "flank" in the name, or "90 percent lean" or leaner)
- Tofu, tempeh, and other foods made with soy, like veggie burgers, tofu dogs, and TVP (textured vegetable protein)
- Beans, such as kidney beans, lentils, chickpeas (garbanzo), white beans (cannellini), black beans, and pinto beans

Soy foods and beans also "count" as carbohydrates, but they are good sources of dietary fiber, which helps to blunt the postmeal glucose response. It does make sense, however, to still keep an eye on the other sources of carbs in the meal (one of the unique challenges for the vegetarian). Beyond hunger and glucose and insulin control, protein plays many important roles in the body and is often neglected, particularly by women trying to lose weight who may see protein foods as "fattening."

Balanced Plate: Step 3

Cover the remaining 25 percent of your plate with a high-quality starch. Despite centuries of understanding about the importance of carbohydrates as a fuel source for the human body, during the low-carb years all types of carbohydrates, including fruit, were deemed "bad" because they "make you fat." I hope you understand by now that single foods don't make you fat. Eating too many calories and not burning them off is what causes weight gain over time. To avoid discarding the good with the bad, we now understand the issue with carbs is about the Two Qs (quality and quantity). For the balanced plate, we've already discussed the advantages of whole grains; specific options will be outlined later in the book (see chapter 10). Allotting one-quarter of a medium-sized plate takes care of the quantity (as long as you abstain from seconds!). If that portion size still seems vague, take your knowledge a step further by learning how to carbohydrate count (the specifics are discussed in chapter 5).

Balanced Plate: Step 4

Include a dab of healthy fat to enhance the flavor and add some healthful nutrients. We now have a balanced plate that accounts for the carbohydrate, protein, and nonstarchy vegetable part of the meal. But what about the fat? Including some fat in cooking or as part of a meal enhances the flavor and texture, helps with absorption of fat-soluble nutrients (vitamins A, D, E, and K and many phytonutrients), helps foods brown during cooking (making it appealing to the eye!), and generally helps us to enjoy our food more. Heart-healthy Mediterranean-diet kinds of fats (olive oil, canola oil, nuts, seeds, and avocado) are good for you if you don't go overboard.

But when it comes to calories, fat is fat. Whether it's good or bad for you, it still has nine calories per gram. Seems like a no-brainer, but I had one client who it actually took me two years to convince that the luscious, heart-healthy extra-virgin olive oil he was lubricating his food with "so it's not dry" was preventing him from losing weight! Try to limit added fat to about two servings per meal. Some examples of *one* serving of fat include the following:

- 1 teaspoon vegetable oil (preferably olive, canola, or peanut oil), butter, or tub margarine (trans-fat-free only)
- 1 tablespoon light margarine (trans-fat-free only)
- 1 tablespoon seeds (sunflower, pumpkin, sesame)
- $1/3$ ounce nuts (for specifics, see the sidebar "Adding Nuts without Going Nuts" in chapter 10)
- 1 tablespoon pine nuts
- $1^1/2$ teaspoons nut butter
- 2 teaspoons tahini (sesame paste)
- 2 teaspoons mayonnaise
- 1 tablespoon reduced-fat mayonnaise
- 1 tablespoon regular salad dressing
- 2 tablespoons reduced-fat salad dressing
- Eight olives
- 2 tablespoons of avocado (one-sixth of a whole avocado)

Remember, we're talking *two servings total* between any oil used in cooking and fats added to foods at the table. Nuts, olives, and avocado are all great additions to a salad (which likely also has dressing)—just watch the quantity. One of the many advantages to cooking at home is that you can control the amount of fat used in preparing the meal. What are the chances the chef in your favorite restaurant is watching how much oil he or she throws in the pan, tosses into the pasta, or mixes into the sauce? No chance at all. Minding your Two Qs requires preparing food at home more and eating out less.

The "Other Carbs"

To account for mealtime extras, the simple approach is to limit fruit intake to one serving at a time, and to have either an eight-ounce glass of milk or a six- to eight-ounce yogurt (plain or light) at a meal or snack, but not both. It is possible to wheel and deal carbs so things aren't this cut-and-dried, but in my experience it works well to suggest eating two to three servings of whole fruit per day, only one at a time. That way your body has only one fruit's worth of sugar to deal with in the hours after your meal or snack. Also, most people can remember, "If I'm having milk with my meal, I'll have my yogurt as a snack." A large portion of something sweet for dessert will lob a lot of sugar into your blood an hour later, while a small portion is more manageable.

Taking Structure to the Next Level with Carbohydrate Counting

For some people simply eating off a smaller plate and following the balanced-plate approach will be enough to curb their carb and calorie intake. But for those who need a tighter rein and more guidance to control their starch portions—or feel completely clueless about portion control of carbohydrates—getting more detailed with carb counting helps set limits. For decades, people with diabetes have been using a great tool, the Exchange Lists for Diabetes, published by the American Diabetes Association (ADA).[6]

In the diabetes exchange lists similar foods are gathered together: starches, fruits, milk/yogurt, sweets/desserts, vegetables, proteins, and fats. The focus for our purposes is on the first four lists—the starches, fruits, milk/yogurt, and sweets/desserts—because those are the only foods that provide significant amounts of carbs. Most vegetables contain very little carbohydrate per serving—they're mostly water and fiber, which is indigestible carbohydrate that doesn't show up as sugar in your blood after digestion. The vegetable list contains those with so little carbohydrate per serving that they're considered a "free food." (The ADA Exchange List recommends three servings of nonstarchy vegetables count as a carb choice, but for the balanced-plate approach they're "free" in any amount. In my more than twenty-two years as a nutritionist, I've yet to see a client overdo it on mixed greens and broccoli!)

Starchy vegetables (like potatoes, corn, peas, and a few others) are listed in the ADA's starch list. Protein foods do not contain carbohydrates, and even though protein foods require some insulin for processing, the effect is not significant. Choices in this group are listed according to fat and calorie content (because of the need to follow a heart-healthy diet and control calories), and lean sources of protein are encouraged. Fats are also listed according to how heart-healthy they are. Saturated and trans fats are discouraged, and monounsaturated and omega-3 fats encouraged. Like protein foods, even though these foods don't require insulin for processing, whether a fat is good or bad for you, they all provide a lot of calories in a small serving. Portion control is key.

Within each exchange list, this system of tracking carbs breaks foods down into portions that would provide a similar amount of carbohydrate, using 15 grams of carbohydrate per portion as their reference. A reasonable "budget" for carbohydrates is 45 to 60 grams per meal and 15 to 30 grams per snack. That way you can decide which carbs you want to eat at a meal or snack and estimate how much you can eat from each source to keep within your carbohydrate budget for that meal or snack. The rest of the calories for your meals and snacks are filled in with nonstarchy vegetables, lean protein choices, and moderate amounts of healthy fats.

We'll delve much deeper into the ins and outs of the exchange lists in chapter 5, on carbohydrate counting.

. . .

Some simple attention to the kinds of carbs you're eating, and choosing low-carb foods to fill up on so you don't eat too much carbohydrate, can make a dent in your calorie intake and insulin response. Looking at the calorie-cutting issue from a different angle—focusing on carb portions and insulin response instead of calorie counting, or diabetes prevention instead of weight loss—can sometimes reinvigorate your motivation to change your diet and start exercising. Same end result, different approach, but maybe with less emotional baggage.

5

The Ins and Outs of Carbohydrate Counting

In addition to using the balanced-plate approach (addressed in chapter 4), carbohydrate counting is another strategy for reshaping your carbohydrate and calorie intake. It's more structured and great for people who need to get a firm grip on portion control; the balanced-plate plan is more general and possibly less intimidating at the outset. In my practice I typically start with the balanced-plate approach and progress to carb counting as the client becomes more comfortable with the concept of portion control. Similar to the fat-gram counting of the 1980s, carb counting is used to help us cap total carb intake for the day. The main difference is that when counting fat grams, we tended not to think about how they were being consumed throughout the day, instead focusing on the daily total. With carb counting, however, we're trying to control the glucose-insulin response that occurs immediately after each meal and snack. The amount of carbohydrate eaten at a meal or snack is what affects our insulin response, so the carb-gram budget has to be broken down and spread out throughout the day.

In chapter 4 we outlined how to figure out your calories for the day, and then how to use that number to calculate your daily carb budget. Breaking that down into meals and snacks will leave most people with 45 to 60 grams of carbohydrate per meal and 15 to 30 grams per snack. All other foods being the same, 45 grams per meal and 15 grams per snack will save you some calories over the 60-gram/30-gram plan. And eating pattern remains important. For most women with PCOS, weight loss is a part of their plan. Losing weight is about eating fewer calories (and burning more through activity). Eating fewer calories requires portion control. Portion control is much easier if you stay ahead of your hunger, eating a reasonably sized meal or snack every three to four hours during the day (and limit your dining out).

So carb counting is as much about distribution as it is about numbers. If you take your daily carb budget, cut it in half, and eat two large meals a day, you're still going to have a glucose-insulin surge in the hours after you eat. What you're really trying to do is control the amount of starch on that quarter of the plate while also keeping an eye on how many other carbs you'll be eating with the meal. The Exchange Lists for Diabetes, published by the American Diabetes Association (ADA), are extremely useful for familiarizing yourself with carbohydrate portions.[1] Similar foods are grouped together into lists: starches, fruits, milk/yogurt, nonstarchy vegetables, proteins and protein substitutes, fats, and sweets/desserts, and other carbohydrates. The Exchange Lists for Diabetes break foods down into lists based on the three major nutrients: carbohydrates, protein (meat and meat substitutes), and fat. They are called exchange lists because each food is listed according to the serving size that would provide roughly the same amount of carbohydrate, protein, fat, and calories in a portion. That way you can "exchange" one serving of food within the same list for another and expect the same blood sugar rise, and subsequent insulin response, regardless of which food you choose.

The starch list includes breads, cereals, rice, pasta, crackers, starchy snack foods, and other types of nontraditional whole grains (like quinoa, barley, amaranth, and bulgur). The starch list also includes starchy vegetables (like beans, peas, lentils, corn, potatoes, sweet potatoes, yams, winter squash, and plantains). The ADA also includes spaghetti sauce in this group because the carbohydrates in tomato sauce are more concentrated than in tomatoes, and there is often added sugar in jarred sauces.

The fruit list includes fresh and canned fruit, dried fruit, and 100 percent fruit juice. The milk list includes milk and yogurt. One percent (low-fat) and nonfat choices are encouraged. The nonstarchy vegetables list includes most fresh vegetables (including salads), frozen and canned vegetables, and tomato and vegetable juices. The meat and meat substitutes list includes animal sources of protein: meat, poultry, seafood, eggs, and cheese. It also includes plant-based protein options: beans, tofu, tempeh,

A Word about Beans

They are great for you! Under no circumstances should you use the fact that they contain carbs as a reason not to eat them. They're one of the highest-fiber foods you can eat, providing both soluble and insoluble fiber; they are a great source of plant protein; and they are a source of many other important nutrients (like iron, B vitamins, magnesium, and potassium). Studies show that eating more plant protein may increase fertility and lower your risk of many chronic diseases. One cup of kidney beans has thirty-seven grams of carbohydrate, but thirteen of those are fiber, which is indigestible and slows down the release of glucose into your blood. That's thirteen grams of great-quality, super-healthy-for-you carbohydrate. So eat them—every day if you can, even if it's only in small quantities thrown into a soup or tossed into a salad, or as a couple of tablespoons of hummus.

soy nuts (edamame), nut butters, and other soy-based foods (like veggie burgers, soy dogs, veggie-nuggets and patties, and soy "crumbles"). Choices are separated into lean, medium-fat, high-fat, and plant-based options.

The fat list includes oils, spreads, nuts and nut butters, seeds, olives, salad dressings, and mayonnaise. Choices are separated into heart-healthy monounsaturated and polyunsaturated fats (which are encouraged) and unhealthy saturated and trans fats (which you're advised to limit or avoid). Alcohol is also addressed in the exchange list, recommending that it be limited to one drink a day for women, two drinks a day for men. Up to this amount of consumption may be associated with some health benefits, although because of the potential negatives associated with alcohol use in some people you should not start drinking alcohol solely for the health benefits. You also need to factor in the calories if you're trying to lose weight. One drink equals 12 ounces of beer, 5 ounces of wine, 1^1/2 ounces of distilled spirits (eighty-proof), or 1 ounce of coffee liqueur.

The sweets, desserts, and other carbohydrates list offers advice on how to work foods with added sugars into your plan by swapping out another source of carbohydrate. Because sweets contain a large amount of carbohydrate in a small portion, suggested portion sizes of sweets—like a 1^1/4-inch-square brownie or a 2-inch-square piece of chocolate cake—are radically small compared to what we're used to. But that's all part of orienting back to reality when it comes to portion control! The exchange lists also include a section on "free foods." These are foods that when limited to the suggested portion will weigh you down with less than twenty calories and no more than five grams of carbohydrate per serving. This allows you to write off small portions of foods that contain sugar but simply don't add up to much when eaten in small amounts—things like a single hard candy, a tablespoon of ketchup, a quarter cup of salsa, or a couple of teaspoons of barbeque sauce.

Animal sources of protein foods do not contain carbohydrates, but many plant-based protein sources (like beans, peas, and hummus) do, counting as both a protein and a carbohydrate. They are great choices, however, so they should be incorporated into your weekly meal plan. You just want to take into account other sources of carbs you may be eating at that meal (for example, eat less rice to make room for the beans, which are a better source of carbohydrate anyway because of the fiber). Even though animal sources of protein foods require some insulin for processing, the effect is not significant. When paired with a carbohydrate, protein helps complicate digestion, slowing down the breakdown of carbohydrates into glucose, thereby blunting your insulin response and leaving you with a more lasting feeling of fullness.

Figuring out Combination Foods

Clearly, not all foods are just a starch, a protein, or vegetable. Casseroles, stews, burritos, and pizza are several food choices wrapped around each other. What to do? Use your best guess, and assume there's probably a little more carbohydrate in the combination food than you think. The American Diabetes Association sells loads of meal-planning guides and cookbooks that break combination foods and recipes down into exchanges on their website (www.diabetes.org). Also, if a recipe provides a nutrient breakdown, you can do the math and see how many fifteen-gram "choices" are in a serving. Here are a few combination foods to give you an idea how this works:

- Five-ounce burrito (bean and beef) equals three starches, one lean meat, and two fats
- One slice cheese pizza ($1/4$ of a 12-inch pizza) equals two starches and two medium-fat meats
- One cup chicken noodle soup equals one carbohydrate
- One cup beef stew equals one starch, one medium-fat meat, and zero to three fats
- Half cup macaroni or pasta salad equals two starches and three fats

The Exchange Lists: Defining a Serving

Let's start with a few important facts that set the foundation for the carbohydrate-counting system. The exchange list system of tracking carbs breaks foods down into portions that would provide a similar amount of carbohydrate, using twelve to fifteen grams of carbohydrate per portion as the reference serving size. A serving of starch or fruit has fifteen grams of carbohydrate, and a serving of milk (any kind) or yogurt (plain or artificially sweetened, called "light" on the label) contains roughly twelve grams of carbohydrate. Because the difference between twelve and fifteen grams of carbohydrate is so small, for simplicity's sake we are going to think along the lines of a milk/yogurt serving containing fifteen grams of carbohydrate. Because the carb content of a serving of starch, fruit, or milk is basically the same, you can interchange a starch, a fruit, or a milk at a meal or snack and consider them all one fifteen-gram carbohydrate choice.

Keep in mind that balance is important, however—to diversify your nutrients you want to be eating carbs from each group every day. Getting used to thinking of carbs in 15-gram carb choices easily fits into our budget of forty-five grams (three choices) to sixty grams (four choices) of carbs per meal, and fifteen grams (one choice) to thirty grams (two choices) of carbs per snack. Remember, if you're really tall or really active, you may need seventy-five grams (five choices) per meal. Starting to think about carbohydrate foods in fifteen-gram carb servings allows you to look at any food label and determine how many carbohydrate serving "equivalents" there are in a serving of any food. For example, if a cereal label lists one serving as having thirty grams of carbohydrate, you'll see that in your head as two carb choices.

Because fiber is nondigestible carbohydrate, according to the American Diabetes Association, if the dietary fiber content is five grams or more, you can subtract *half* that number from the total carbs listed on the label.[2] For example, if a cereal has thirty grams of carb in a serving, but six of it is fiber, then you "count" the serving as having twenty-seven grams of carb, or slightly less than two carb choices. In addition to high-fiber foods being all-around healthy choices, having five or more grams of fiber in a food may help slow down the absorption of the other carbs in that food, blunting the insulin response. Once you begin to view carbohydrates in fifteen-gram carb units, you can decide which carbs you want to eat at a meal or snack and estimate how much you can eat of those foods to keep within your carb budget. Although this doesn't need to happen every single time you eat, keep in mind the benefits of pairing carbohydrates with protein, and a little bit of healthy fat if possible, to blunt the postmeal insulin response and help you feel fuller longer. The 80/20 rule applies pretty well here—aim to pair your carbs with protein 80 percent of the time so that what happens 20 percent of the time doesn't matter as much.

Before we move on, let's be clear about one thing: by no means is carb counting meant to rationalize eating sixty grams of "junk food" carbs in place of food that does your body good. A twenty-ounce cola has sixty-five grams of carbohydrate in it, but that doesn't mean it's okay to let such a nutrient-poor food gobble up so much of your budget! If you're going to budget in some sweets, it's best to cut back a little on your healthy carbs to make room for a small amount of a special treat on occasion.

Portion Control: Learning by Measuring

To accurately estimate the amount of carbohydrate (and calories) you're eating, knowledge of portion sizes is critical. Assume that you don't know exactly what a cup of cereal or a third of a cup of cooked rice looks like. If you don't have any, go out and buy a set of dry measuring cups, a liquid measuring cup that holds up to two cups, and a set of measuring spoons. It's also not a bad idea to get a food scale. Fancy, more expensive scales can be found in cooking stores, but a cheap ten-dollar postage or utility scale may work just as well. All around us, portion sizes have been expanding over the past twenty years. If you're over forty, you may remember when all fast-food burgers were the size of a children's meal, and when a soda bottle was eight ounces. But even then, you're likely to be as prone as anyone to underestimate portions of food, mostly because we're not genetically hardwired to resist eating what we see. Studies show that the larger a portion of food, the more people tend to underestimate its calories. So don't guess initially, even if you think you know. Measure foods a few times so that you can accurately eyeball serving sizes. Then occasionally go back and measure again to see if your portion sizes have grown ("portion creep" is very common!).

The Exchange Lists: Planning Your Plate

Remember, you want to focus on the first four lists—starches, fruits, milk/yogurt, and sweets/desserts—to control your carbs. They are the carb-containing foods. The last three lists—nonstarchy vegetables, proteins, and fats—are there to help you make healthy choices from these groups to control your calorie and fat intake. These are the foods that help you walk away from a meal still feeling full without ramping up your insulin response.

The Starch List

Cereals, grains, pasta, breads, crackers, snacks, starchy vegetables, and cooked beans, peas, and lentils are starches. In general, one starch is

- Half cup cooked cereal, grain, or starchy vegetable
- $^1/_3$ cup cooked rice or pasta
- 1 ounce (30 grams) bread product, such as one regular-size slice of bread
- $^3/_4$ to 1 ounce most snack foods

Things to consider: A choice on the starch list has 15 grams of carbohydrate, 0 to 3 grams of protein, 0 to 1 grams of fat, and 80 calories. Choose low-fat starches as often as possible. When choosing dense starches like bagels and large rolls, be sure to check out how much it weighs. Each ounce *by weight* (30 grams) is one starch choice. Many bagels are four ounces—or four starch choices! An open handful is about one cup or one to two ounces of a snack food. For maximum health benefits, eat three or more servings of whole grains each day.

The Starch List

FOOD	SERVING SIZE
BREAD	
Bagel, large (about 4 ounces)	$^1/_4$ bagel (1 ounce)
Biscuit, $2^1/_2$-inch diameter	1
Bread	
Reduced calorie	2 slices
White, whole grain, pumpernickel, rye, unfrosted raisin	1 slice (1 ounce)
Chapatti, small (6-inch diameter)	1

The Starch List, continued

FOOD	SERVING SIZE
Cornbread, 1³/₄-inch cube	1 (1¹/₂ ounces)
English muffin	¹/₂ (1 ounce)
Hot dog or hamburger bun	¹/₂ (1 ounce)
Naan bread (8-inch diameter)	¹/₄ piece
Pancake (4-inch diameter)	1
Pita (6-inch diameter)	¹/₂ pita
Roll, small, plain	1 (1 ounce)
Stuffing, bread	¹/₃ cup (higher-fat choice)
Taco shell (5-inch diameter)	2 (higher-fat choice)
Tortilla, corn or flour (6-inch diameter)	1
Tortilla, flour (10-inch diameter)	¹/₃
Waffle (4-inch square)	1 (opt for whole grain, higher-fat choice)
CEREALS AND GRAINS	
Barley, cooked	¹/₃ cup
Bran, dry	
Oat	¹/₄ cup
Wheat	¹/₂ cup
Bulgur (cooked)	¹/₂ cup
Cereals	
Bran	¹/₂ cup
Cooked (oats, oatmeal)	¹/₂ cup
Puffed	1¹/₂ cups
Shredded wheat, plain	¹/₂ cup
Sugar coated	¹/₂ cup
Unsweetened, ready-to-eat	³/₄ cup
Couscous	¹/₃ cup
Granola	
Low-fat	¹/₄ cup
Regular	¹/₄ cup (higher-fat choice)
Grits, cooked	¹/₂ cup
Kasha	¹/₂ cup
Millet, cooked	¹/₃ cup
Muesli	¹/₄ cup
Pasta, cooked	¹/₃ cup
Polenta, cooked	¹/₃ cup
Quinoa, cooked	¹/₃ cup

The Starch List, continued

FOOD	SERVING SIZE
Rice, white or brown, cooked	1/3 cup
Tabouli, prepared	1/2 cup
Wheat germ, dry	3 tablespoons
Wild rice, cooked	1/2 cup
STARCHY VEGETABLES	
Cassava	1/3 cup
Corn	1/2 cup kernels or 1/2 large cob
Hominy, canned	3/4 cup
Mixed vegetables with corn, peas, or pasta	1 cup
Parsnips	1/2 cup
Peas, green	1/2 cup
Plantain, ripe	1/3 cup
Potato	
Baked with skin	1/4 large (3 ounces)
Boiled, all kinds	1/2 cup or 1/2 medium
Mashed with milk and fat	1/2 cup
French fried (oven baked)	1 cup (2 ounces)
Pumpkin, canned, no sugar added	1 cup
Spaghetti with pasta sauce	1/2 cup
Squash (winter, acorn, butternut)	1 cup
Succotash	1/2 cup
Yam, sweet potato, plain	1/2 cup
CRACKERS AND SNACKS	
Crackers	
Round-butter type	6
Animal crackers	8
Saltine-type	6
Sandwich-style, cheese or peanut butter filling	3
Whole wheat regular	2–5 (3/4 ounce)
Whole wheat crisp breads	2–5 (3/4 ounce)
Graham cracker	3 (2 1/2-inch squares)
Matzo	3/4 ounce
Melba toast, about 2-inch by 4-inch piece	4 pieces
Oyster crackers	20

The Starch List, continued

FOOD	SERVING SIZE
Popcorn	3 cups
Pretzels	3/4 ounce
Rice cakes (4-inch diameter)	2
Snack chips	
Fat-free or baked (tortilla, potato), baked pita chips	15–20 (3/4 ounce)
Regular (tortilla, potato)	9–13 (3/4 ounce)
BEANS, PEAS, AND LENTILS *(Note: The choices on this list count as one starch and one lean meat.)*	
Baked beans	1/3 cup
Beans, cooked (black, pinto, garbanzo, kidney, lima, navy, white)	1/2 cup
Lentils, cooked (brown, yellow, green)	1/2 cup
Peas, cooked (black eyed, split)	1/2 cup
Refried beans, canned (look for fat-free)	1/2 cup

The Fruit List

Fruit can be fresh, frozen, canned, or 100 percent fruit juice. A serving of fruit is

- 1/2 cup of canned fruit or fruit salad
- 1/2 cup of unsweetened fruit juice
- 1 small fruit (4 ounces)
- 2 tablespoons of dried fruit

Things to consider: A choice on the fruit list has 15 grams of carb, 0 protein, 0 fat, and 60 calories. Limit your juice to one serving or less per day, as juice has no fiber. Fresh fruit is preferable whenever possible. Aim for a minimum of two fruits daily, but eat them separately. Think of dried fruit as something you sprinkle on or mix into something, as it's easy to go overboard when you eat it alone. Avoid fruits canned in heavy syrup. Look for canned fruits that say "extra light syrup," "no sugar added," or "juice packed."

The Fruit List

FRUIT	SERVING SIZE
Apple, unpeeled, small	1 (4 ounces)
Apples, dried	4 rings
Applesauce, unsweetened	1/2 cup
Apricots	
Canned	1/2 cup
Dried	8 halves
Fresh	4 whole
Banana, extra small	1 (4 ounces)
Blackberries	3/4 cup
Blueberries	3/4 cup
Cantaloupe, small	1/3 melon or 2 cups cubed
Cherries	
Sweet, canned	1/2 cup
Sweet fresh	12
Dates	3
Dried fruits (blueberries, cherries, cranberries, mixed fruit, raisins)	2 tablespoons
Figs	
Dried	1 1/2
Fresh	1 1/2 large or 2 medium (3 1/2 ounces)
Fruit cocktail	1/2 cup
Grapefruit	
Large	1/2 (11 ounces)
Sections, canned	3/4 cup
Grapes, small	17 (3 ounces)
Honeydew melon	1 slice or 1 cup cubed (10 ounces)
Kiwi	1 (3 1/2 ounces)
Mandarin oranges, canned	3/4 cup
Mango, small	1/2 fruit (5 1/2 ounces) or 1/2 cup
Nectarine, small	1 (5 ounces)
Orange, small	1 (6 ounces)
Papaya	1/2 fruit or 1 cup cubed (8 ounces)
Peaches	
Canned	1/2 cup
Fresh, medium	1 (6 ounces)

The Fruit List, continued

FRUIT	SERVING SIZE
Pears	
Canned	1/2 cup
Fresh, large	1/2 (4 ounces)
Pineapple	
Canned	1/2 cup
Fresh	3/4 cup
Plums	
Canned	1/2 cup
Dried (prunes)	3
Small	2 (5 ounces)
Raspberries	1 cup
Strawberries	1 1/4 cups whole berries
Tangerines, small	2 (8 ounces)
Watermelon	1 slice or 1 1/4 cups cubed (13 1/2 ounces)
JUICES	
Apple juice/cider	1/2 cup
Fruit juice blends, 100 percent juice	1/3 cup
Grape juice	1/3 cup
Grapefruit juice	1/2 cup
Orange juice	1/2 cup
Pineapple juice	1/2 cup
Prune juice	1/3 cup

The Milk List

This list includes milk and yogurt. An important note: Cheese is on the protein list. In general, a serving is one cup of milk, or eight ounces of plain yogurt, or six ounces of flavored yogurt.

Things to consider: One milk serving is 12 grams of carbohydrate, 8 grams of protein, and 0 to 8 grams of fat. To keep things easy, for our purposes we are going to round one milk serving up to 15 grams of carb to be consistent with our other two carb groups (starches and fruits). Opt for 1 percent (low-fat) or nonfat milk. Two percent milk is only slightly lower in fat than whole milk. If you use flavorings in milk that are not artificially sweetened, it will use up one of your carb choices at that meal (you have to count the extra carbs). Yogurt should be artificially sweetened or it will also use up one of your carb choices at that meal. Some flavored Greek yogurts have less added sugar. Compare labels.

The Milk List

FOOD	SERVING SIZE
MILK AND YOGURT	
Fat-free or 1 percent low-fat milk	1 cup
Evaporated milk	$\frac{1}{2}$ cup
Yogurt, plain nonfat or 1 percent	8 ounces
Yogurt, flavored with artificial sweetener	6 ounces
Milk, buttermilk, goat's milk	1 cup
Evaporated milk	$\frac{1}{2}$ cup
Chocolate milk (sugar-free, fat-free, or 1 percent)	1 cup
Eggnog	$\frac{1}{2}$ cup
Rice milk (fat-free or low-fat)	1 cup
Soy milk (unflavored)	1 cup

The Sweets, Desserts, and Other Carbohydrates List

You can substitute a choice from this list for other carbohydrates from the starch, fruit, or milk lists, even though these foods contain added sugars. Each carb choice is 15 grams of carb. It's critically important to be portion conscious, however, as the carbs from sweets add up quickly. Set a goal of limiting sweets to special occasions, particularly if "just one" tends to lead to "many." Remember, for physiological reasons, the more you indulge in sweets, the more you'll want them. This list highlights how many carb choices are gobbled up by a serving.

The Sweets, Desserts, and Other Carbohydrates List

FOOD	SERVING SIZE	CARB CHOICES
BEVERAGES		
Energy drink	8 ounces	2 carbs
Fruit drink or lemonade	8 ounces	2 carbs
Hot chocolate (regular or sugar-free)	8 ounces	1 carb
Sports drink	8 ounces	1 carb

The Sweets, Desserts, and Other Carbohydrates List, continued

FOOD	SERVING SIZE	CARB CHOICES
DESSERTS		
Brownie, small	1¼-inch square	1 carb
Cake		
Angel food, unfrosted	1 slice (¹⁄₁₂ of cake)	2 carbs
Frosted	2-inch square	2 carbs
Unfrosted	2-inch square	1 carb
Cookies		
Chocolate chip	2 (2½ inches across)	1 carb
Gingersnap	3 cookies	1 carb
Sandwich with creme filling	2 small	1 carb
Sugar-free	3 small or 1 large	1 carb
Vanilla wafer	5 cookies	1 carb
Cupcakes, frosted	1 small	2 carbs
Fruit cobbler	½ cup	3 carbs
Gelatin, regular	½ cup	1 carb (sugar-free gelatin is free)
Pie		
Fruit (double crust)	1 slice (¹⁄₆ of 8-inch pie)	3 carbs
Pumpkin or custard	1 slice (¹⁄₆ of 8-inch pie)	1½ carbs
Pudding		
Regular	½ cup	2 carbs
Sugar-free	½ cup	1 carb
CANDY, SWEETS, SWEETENERS		
Candy bar, chocolate/peanut	2 "fun size" bars (1 ounce)	1½ carbs
Candy, hard	3 pieces	1 carb
Chocolate "kisses"	5 pieces	1 carb
Fruit snacks, chewy	1 roll	1 carb
Fruit spread, 100 percent fruit	1½ tablespoons	1 carb
Honey	1 tablespoon	1 carb
Jam or jelly	1 tablespoon	1 carb
Sugar	1 tablespoon	1 carb
Syrup (chocolate, regular maple)	1 tablespoon	1 carb
Syrup, light	2 tablespoons	1 carb
CONDIMENTS AND SAUCES		
Barbeque sauce	3 tablespoons	1 carb
Cranberry sauce	¼ cup	1½ carbs

The Sweets, Desserts, and Other Carbohydrates List, continued

FOOD	SERVING SIZE	CARB CHOICES
Salad dressing, fat-free, low-fat, cream-based	3 tablespoons	1 carb
Sweet and sour sauce	3 tablespoons	1 carb
DOUGHNUTS, MUFFINS, AND PASTRIES		
Banana nut bread	1-inch slice	2 carbs
Doughnut		
Plain	1 medium	1½ carbs
Glazed	3¼ inches across	2 carbs
Muffin (4 ounces)	¼ muffin	1 carb
Danish	1 (2½ ounces)	2½ carbs
FROZEN DESSERTS		
Frozen pop	1	½ carb
Fruit juice bars, 100 percent fruit juice	1 bar	1 carb
Ice cream		
Fat-free	½ cup	1½ carbs
Light and no sugar added	½ cup	1 carb
Regular	½ cup	1 carb (high in fat and calories)
Sherbet and sorbet	½ cup	2 carbs
Frozen yogurt, fat-free and regular	½ cup	1 carb
GRANOLA BARS, MEAL REPLACEMENT BARS, TRAIL MIX		
Granola bar, regular or low-fat	1 bar (1 ounce)	1½ carbs
Meal replacement bar	1 bar (2 ounces)	2 carbs
Trail mix	1 ounce	1 carb

The Nonstarchy Vegetables List

All the vegetables on this list are so low in carbohydrates that we consider them a free food. Following the balanced-plate approach, your goal is to cover half your plate with nonstarchy vegetables. If necessary, start with a third of the plate and work your way up. A serving of nonstarchy vegetables is ½ cup of cooked vegetables or vegetable juice or 1 cup of raw vegetables.

Things to consider: A serving of nonstarchy vegetables contains only five grams of carb, two grams of protein, and twenty-five calories. Try to include at least a half cup cooked or a cup raw vegetables with lunch, and a cup cooked or two cups raw vegetables with dinner. Look for a variety of colors in the vegetables you're eating. Different-colored vegetables offer different nutrients. Be sure not to load your vegetables down with a lot of fat. Every teaspoon of butter or tub margarine adds forty calories. Remember that corn, peas, potatoes, sweet potatoes, winter squash, and beans are on the starch list.

The Nonstarchy Vegetables List

Artichoke	Asparagus	Baby corn
Bamboo shoots	Beans (green, wax, Italian)	Bean sprouts
Beets	Borscht	Broccoli
Brussels sprouts	Cabbage	Carrots
Cauliflower	Celery	Coleslaw (no dressing)
Cucumber	Eggplant	Green onions or scallions
Greens (collard, kale, mustard, turnip)	Hearts of palm	Jicama
Kohlrabi	Leeks	Lettuce (carb content is so low that all varieties are considered free)
Mixed vegetables (without corn, peas, or pasta)	Mung bean sprouts	Mushrooms
Okra	Onions	Pea pods
Peppers, all varieties	Radishes	Rutabaga
Sauerkraut	Spinach	Squash (summer, zucchini)
Swiss chard	Tomatoes	Tomato sauce
Tomato/vegetable juice	Turnips	Water chestnuts

The Meat and Meat Substitutes List

The key to being able to eat a diet a little higher in protein without eating too much unhealthful saturated fat is to choose lean sources of protein, with few exceptions. Because protein is found in so many different foods, serving sizes vary.

Things to consider: In general, a protein choice has no carbs (unless it's a plant protein), seven grams of protein, and three to eight or more grams of fat. Calories per protein choice range from forty-five to a hundred calories or more per serving, depending on fat content. For meat, poultry, or seafood, a choice is *one ounce cooked*, but you would portion out three to four ounces at a meal. Three ounces is about the size of a deck of cards, and four ounces is about the size of a hockey puck. A snack may include one to two protein choices.

Protein choices can be lean (zero to three grams of fat per ounce), medium-fat (four to seven grams of fat per ounce), high-fat (more than eight grams of fat per ounce), or plant-based (the amount of fat varies). Try to choose proteins with five grams of fat or less per ounce. The only protein foods that contain carbs are the plant-based proteins. If the amount of plant protein you're eating contains close to fifteen grams of carb, count it as a carb and a protein, but give yourself a little wiggle room if you're not diabetic. Choose poultry, seafood, or plant-based proteins whenever possible. If you eat meat, opt for lean select or choice cuts that have the word "loin," "round," or "flank" in the name, or are 90 percent lean or leaner. Bake, roast, broil, grill, poach, steam, or boil instead of frying your proteins, and trim off visible fat.

The Meat and Meat Substitutes List

FOOD	SERVING SIZE
LEAN MEATS AND MEAT SUBSTITUTES (45 CALORIES PER OUNCE)	
Beef, lean cuts trimmed of fat	1 ounce
Cheese with 3 grams of fat	1 ounce
Cottage cheese	1/4 cup
Egg substitutes	1/4 cup
Egg whites	2
Fish, any kind	1 ounce
Game: buffalo, venison, and so on	1 ounce
Lamb: chop, leg, or roast	1 ounce
Oysters	6 medium
Pork, lean: Canadian bacon, rib or loin chop/roast, ham, tenderloin	1 ounce
Poultry without the skin	1 ounce
Salmon, canned	1 ounce
Sardines, canned	2 small
Sausages with 3 grams of fat or less per ounce	1 ounce
Shellfish: clams, crab, lobster, scallops, shrimp	1 ounce
Tuna canned with water, drained	1 ounce
Veal: loin, chop, roast	1 ounce

The Meat and Meat Substitutes List, continued

FOOD	SERVING SIZE
MEDIUM-FAT MEAT AND MEAT SUBSTITUTES (75 calories per ounce)	
Beef: corned beef, ground beef, prime grades trimmed of fat (prime rib), short ribs	1 ounce
Cheeses with 4 to 7 grams of fat per ounce	1 ounce
Egg	1
Fish, fried	1 ounce
Lamb: ground, rib roast	1 ounce
Pork: cutlet, shoulder roast	1 ounce
Poultry: chicken with skin, fried chicken, ground turkey	1 ounce
Ricotta cheese	1/4 cup
Sausage with 4 to 7 grams fat per ounce	1 ounce
Veal, cutlet (no breading)	1 ounce
HIGH-FAT MEAT AND MEAT SUBSTITUTES (try to eat three or fewer servings per week; these are 100 calories or more per ounce)	
Bacon	
Pork	2 slices
Turkey	2 slices
Cheese: regular American, blue, Brie, Cheddar, hard goat, Monterey Jack, queso, and Swiss	1 ounce
Hot dog: beef, pork, or combination (10 per 1-pound package)	1
Hot dog: turkey, chicken (10 per 1-pound package)	1
Pork: ground, sausage, spareribs	1 ounce
Processed sandwich meats with 8 grams of fat or more: bologna, hard salami, pastrami	1 ounce
Sausage with 8 grams of fat or more per ounce: bratwurst, chorizo, Italian, knockwurst, smoked, summer	1 ounce
PLANT-BASED PROTEINS (these contain some carbohydrates but much of it is fiber; calories vary)	
Soy-based "bacon" strips	3
Baked beans	1/3 cup
Beans, cooked: black, garbanzo, kidney, lima, navy, pinto, white	1/2 cup
"Beef" or "sausage" crumbles, soy-based	2 ounces
"Chicken" nuggets, soy-based	2 (1 1/2 ounces)
Edamame	1/2 cup
Falafel (spiced chickpeas and wheat patties)	3 patties (2-inch diameter)
Hot dog, soy-based	1
Hummus	1/3 cup

The Meat and Meat Substitutes List, continued

FOOD	SERVING SIZE
Lentils, brown, green, or yellow	1/2 cup
Meatless burger, soy-based	3 ounces
Meatless burger, vegetable- and starch-based	1
Nut spreads: almond butter, cashew butter, peanut butter, soy nut butter	1 tablespoon
Peas, cooked: black-eyed and split peas	1/2 cup
Refried beans, canned	1/2 cup
"Sausage" patties, soy-based	1
Soy nuts, unsalted	3/4 ounce
Tempeh	1/4 cup
Tofu	4 ounces (1/2 cup)
Tofu, light	4 ounces (1/2 cup)

The Fats List

Fats can be either good for you (in moderation) or bad for you. Healthy fats are monounsaturated fats (they can help lower cholesterol and raise healthy HDL), omega-3s (these are anti-inflammatory, can lower triglyceride levels and risk of heart disease), and polyunsaturated (these can help lower cholesterol). "Bad fats" are saturated fats (they raise unhealthy LDL cholesterol and are solid at room temperature) and trans fats (these raise cholesterol levels and are mostly artificially made via hydrogenated and partially hydrogenated fats). Things to consider:

- A fat choice is based on a serving that has five grams of total fat.
- Fats and oils are mixtures of several different types of fat. The predominant fat dictates which list it's in.
- The idea is to replace saturated fats with healthy fats, not to add healthy fat without taking away the unhealthy fat.
- All fat has the same number of calories—nine calories per gram! Too many calories consumed that aren't burned off will cause weight gain regardless of the source.
- When choosing a spread, look carefully at food labels. Liquid vegetable oil should be the first ingredient listed in regular tub spread

and the second ingredient after water in light spreads. All should be trans-fat-free.

- A tablespoon is about the size of your thumb, and a teaspoon about the size of your thumb tip.

Nut Note

The American Diabetes Association counts nuts as fats in small portions (see "The Fats List" below), but counts 1 tablespoon of nut butter as a protein even though it contains only 3½ grams of protein (a standard protein choice has 7 grams protein). With snacks, for our purposes, we will do the same with nuts: count half ounce of nuts as a protein choice even though a half ounce averages only about 2 to 3 grams of protein. When a half ounce of nuts is eaten with a carb (for example, half ounce of walnuts and a pear) as part of a snack, both the protein and fat lend a sense of fullness and satisfaction to the snack.

The Fats List

FOOD	SERVING SIZE
MONOUNSATURATED FATS	
Avocado, medium	2 tablespoons
Nut butters: almond, cashew, peanut	1½ teaspoons
Nuts	
Almonds	6
Brazil	2
Cashews	6
Hazelnuts	5
Macadamia	3
Mixed	6
Peanuts	10
Pecans	4 halves
Pistachios	16
Oil: canola, olive, peanut	1 teaspoon
Olives	
Black	8 large
Green	10 large

The Fats List, continued

FOOD	SERVING SIZE
POLYUNSATURATED FATS	
Margarine: lower-fat, trans-fat-free	1 tablespoon
Margarine: tub or stick, trans-fat-free	1 teaspoon
Mayonnaise	
Reduced fat	1 tablespoon
Regular	1 teaspoon
Mayonnaise-style salad dressing	
Reduced fat	1 tablespoon
Regular	2 teaspoons
Nuts	
Pine nuts	1 tablespoon
Walnuts	4 halves
Oil: corn, cottonseed, flaxseed, grape seed, safflower, soybean, sunflower	1 teaspoon
Plant stanol spreads (Benecol)	
Light	1 tablespoon
Regular	2 teaspoon
Salad dressing (fat-free is on the Sweets list)	
Reduced fat	2 tablespoons
Regular	1 tablespoon
Seeds	
Flaxseed, whole	1 tablespoon
Pumpkin, sunflower	1 tablespoon
Sesame seeds	1 tablespoon
Tahini or sesame paste	2 teaspoons
SATURATED FATS	
Bacon, cooked, regular or turkey	1 slice (in larger portion is a fatty meat)
Butter	
Reduced fat	1 tablespoon
Stick	1 teaspoon
Whipped	2 teaspoons
Coconut, sweetened, shredded	2 tablespoons
Coconut milk	
Light	1/3 cup
Regular	1 1/2 tablespoons

The Fats List, continued

FOOD	SERVING SIZE
Cream	
Half-and-half	2 tablespoons
Heavy	1 tablespoon
Light	1¹/₂ tablespoons
Whipped	2 tablespoons
Whipped, pressurized	¹/₄ cup
Cream cheese	
Reduced fat	1¹/₂ tablespoons
Regular	1 tablespoon
Lard	1 teaspoon
Oil: coconut, palm, palm kernel	1 teaspoon
Salt pork	¹/₄ ounce
Shortening, solid	1 teaspoon
Sour cream	
Reduced fat or light	3 tablespoons
Regular	2 tablespoons

The Free Foods List

These foods contain fewer than twenty calories and five grams of carb in the serving size shown. Eaten in this amount, these foods are considered "free." Take note, however: In larger portions they may start to add up to the point where you need to count them in your budget or factor in their calories. The idea is to not sweat the small stuff, but to be realistic about how much you're eating.

The Free Foods List

FOOD	SERVING SIZE
Barbecue sauce	2 teaspoons
Candy, hard (regular or sugar-free)	1 piece
Cream cheese, fat-free	1 tablespoon
Creamers	
Nondairy, liquid	1 tablespoon
Nondairy, powdered	2 teaspoons
Gelatin, sugar-free	unlimited

The Free Foods List, continued

FOOD	SERVING SIZE
Gum (preferably sugar-free)	unlimited
Honey mustard	1 tablespoon
Horseradish	unlimited
Jam or jelly, light or no added sugar	2 teaspoons
Ketchup	1 tablespoon
Lemon juice	unlimited
Margarine spread	
Fat-free	1 tablespoon
Reduced fat	1 teaspoon
Mayonnaise	
Fat-free	1 tablespoon
Reduced fat	1 teaspoon
Miso	1¹/₂ teaspoons
Mustard	unlimited
Parmesan cheese, grated	1 tablespoon
Pickles	
Dill	1¹/₂ medium
Sweet, bread and butter	2 slices
Sweet, gherkin	³/₄ ounce
Relish	1 tablespoon
Salad dressing	
Fat-free or low-fat	1 tablespoon
Fat-free Italian	2 tablespoons
Salsa	¹/₄ cup
Sour cream, fat-free or reduced fat	1 tablespoon
Soy sauce, light or regular	1 tablespoon
Sweet and sour sauce	2 teaspoons
Sweet chili sauce	2 teaspoons
Syrup, sugar-free	2 tablespoons
Taco sauce	1 tablespoon
Vinegar	unlimited
Whipped topping	
Light or fat-free	2 tablespoons
Regular	1 tablespoon
Yogurt, any type	2 tablespoons

The Free Foods List, continued

FOOD	SERVING SIZE
FREE DRINKS AND MIXES	
Carbonated water	any moderate amount
Club soda	any moderate amount
Cocoa powder, unsweetened (1 tablespoon)	any moderate amount
Coffee or tea, unsweetened or with sugar substitute	any moderate amount
Diet soft drinks	any moderate amount
Sugar-free drink mixes	any moderate amount
Tonic water, diet	any moderate amount
Water, flavored, carbohydrate-free	any moderate amount

Other Ingredients Not to Worry About

There are many other ingredients you can consider "free foods." These include flavoring extracts, garlic, herbs, spices, nonstick cooking spray, hot pepper sauce, cooking wine, and Worcestershire sauce. Note: Beware seasonings that contain salt!

Using the Exchange Lists: Let's Do Dinner!

Now that you have your lists of carb-containing foods and serving/portion sizes, you can start using your carbohydrate budget to control the amount of carbs you eat at a meal or snack. Remember, the ultimate goal of either approach you choose (the balanced-plate or the exchange-list system) is to help you better understand what a reasonable amount of carbohydrate intake is for someone with insulin resistance. But eating smaller portions of carbs and spreading them out over the day is also going to help you weed some calories out of your diet—as long as you don't compensate by eating excessive amounts of protein foods or too much added fat to pick up the slack. It's not called the balanced plate for nothing: you want enough protein to meet your nutrition needs and help fill you up; enough healthy fat to meet your needs for fat-soluble nutrients and make your food taste good; and a lot of plant foods to ramp up your intake of fiber and health-promoting nutrients and to take up a lot of space on your plate and in your stomach so that it's easier not to overdose on carbs.

As tempting as it may be, don't overrestrict carbs either. You'll then be "dieting" (practicing an unsustainable behavior), which may trigger reactive overeating later. Begin with a reasonably sized plate. Portion out a three- to four-ounce portion of protein to cover roughly 25 percent of your plate. Now cover half the plate with nonstarchy vegetables. It can be a large portion of a cooked vegetable, a large salad with ideally at least five different ingredients (to really diversify the nutrients and make the salad more filling), or one portion of a cooked vegetable and a small salad with at least three ingredients. This leaves us with the carbohydrate piece to figure out. Let's start with the starch. If you look at the starch list, one option is a third cup of cooked brown rice, which is fifteen grams of carbohydrate or one carb choice. You have at a minimum forty-five grams of carbohydrate to work with, so depending on what other carbs you eat at that meal, you may be able to eat two portions of rice (two-thirds' cup)—or thirty grams of carbs.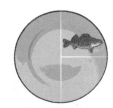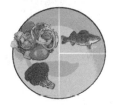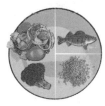

Let's assume you're going with one serving of rice, which populates the remaining quarter of the plate. You've now used up fifteen grams of your forty-five-gram carb budget, leaving you with thirty grams to "spend" throughout the rest of your meal; if you have a sixty-gram carb budget, you can go for that two servings of brown rice and still be left with thirty grams of carbohydrate. If you add an eight-ounce glass of 1 percent milk (one carb choice) and a cup of cantaloupe cubes (one carb choice), you've hit your budget of roughly forty-five grams of carbohydrate for the meal.

If you've already eaten your recommended minimum of two fruits on 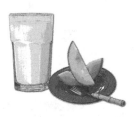 this day, you may decide to spend fifteen grams of carbohydrate on a dessert instead of a fruit, maybe half a cup of low-fat ice cream. This is how you work in your "special treats." Limit how often you decide to spend a chunk of your carb budget on foods without nutritional value, however. A big part of the

benefit you get from eating better is the positive feedback you get from your body for filling it with good-
quality food, which is unlikely to happen with too
much processed food, even if it doesn't deliver a lot
of carbohydrate. Let's look at some other examples of
carb-controlled meals.

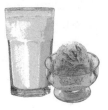

Carb-Controlled Meals

45-GRAM CARB BUDGET	60-GRAM CARB BUDGET
3–4 ounces grilled chicken	3–4 ounces grilled chicken
1/2 cup mashed potato (1 choice)	1 cup mashed potato (2 choices)
1 cup broccoli	1 cup broccoli
Salad with 1–2 tablespoons low-fat dressing	Salad with 1–2 tablespoons low-fat dressing
8 ounces of 1 percent milk (1 choice)	8 ounces of skim milk (1 choice)
1 medium orange (1 choice)	1 1/4 cups sliced strawberries (1 choice)

Either of these meals could be adjusted by using the exchange lists
to make alternative choices. The three- to four-ounce portion of chicken
could be swapped out for a same-size portion of turkey, fish, lean meat,
tofu, or other protein choice. The vegetables are nonstarchy, so we don't
count their carbs toward our total carb budget. Any vegetable or salad
listed as nonstarchy in the exchange lists is considered a freebie unless it's
fried or loaded with butter, cream, or cheese sauce. The starch choice can
be swapped out for any other serving of starch from the starch list—one
serving in the forty-five-gram budget and two servings in the sixty-gram
budget. It could be brown rice, couscous, pasta (preferably whole wheat
pasta or at least one of the pasta blends, like Barilla Plus), sweet potato,
winter squash, corn, or peas. It's your choice.

The carb content of milk doesn't change with the fat content, so either
skim or 1 percent milk is a healthy choice. Two percent milk is very close
to whole milk, which is about 3.25 percent milk fat, so those who like
thicker milk should opt for one of the enriched low-fat or fat-free milks,
like Over the Moon (available nationwide) and Hood's Simply Smart (in
the Northeast), to control their fat and calorie intake. The fruit choice
could be any of the fresh, canned, or dried options in the fruit list. Juice
should be limited to around a third to half cup at breakfast. Opt for whole

fruit choices the rest of the day. This is primarily because juice is a lot easier to go overboard on than whole fruit—one medium-sized fresh fruit has the same calories as only about a half cup of fruit juice. Liquid calories, like those from juice, also don't contribute to a feeling of fullness the way whole fruit does.

Be Wary of Bread

Most people love bread in one form or another. Bread is not the evil enemy. Instead of fretting about overdosing on bread carbs, just use the Two Qs to steer you in the right direction. It's about the *quality* (whole grain breads, muffins, rolls, bagels, tortillas, over white flour options) and the *quantity* (you have to include them in your carb budget). As a general rule, I suggest not eating bread with a meal unless it *is* the carb, as in a sandwich with lunch, a whole wheat English muffin with breakfast, or as one slice toasted with reduced-fat cheese or a thin layer of peanut butter for a snack. You want to avoid already having a carb planned for the meal and then eating bread on top of that. For example, one way to enjoy bread without guilt at dinner is to have it as *the* starch choice. In our house we love good-quality bread, so every other week or so we'll have for dinner a hearty, protein-dense salad with the bread as the starch. That way we're not eating bread as added carbs and calories—there's no reason not to enjoy it.

It is possible to have one serving of starch, like a third of a cup of brown rice, for example, and enjoy a slice of bread as your second carb choice, but you need to be well aware of whether you can stop at just one slice! Another note about bread: One of the positive benefits of the low-carb craze was an increased awareness of the difference between white bread and whole grain bread. My shopping list (see chapter 11) directs you to buy breads that ideally are made of 100 percent whole grains with two to three grams of fiber per slice. Calories matter, however, and a slice of bread should weigh roughly one ounce and contain around 80 to 90 calories. Some breads have two to three grams of fiber but at a cost of 120 to 150 calories per slice! When reading bread labels, look at three things: (1) the first ingredient ideally should be 100 percent whole grain flour, (2) the fiber should be two to three grams per slice, and (3) the calories should be in the 80- to 90-calorie range.

What about Lunch?

Same rules, different meal. These examples show one sandwich meal and one salad-based lunch.

Lunch: Sandwich or Salad?

45-GRAM CARB BUDGET	60-GRAM CARB BUDGET
3 ounces turkey or 2 ounces turkey and 1 ounce cheese	3 ounces grilled chicken
Mustard or low-fat mayonnaise	Low-fat salad dressing
Half a 6-inch whole wheat pita (1 choice)	6-inch whole wheat pita (2 choices)
Lettuce and tomato	Lettuce, tomato, cucumber, peppers, onions
Baby carrots dipped in low-fat dressing	Carrots, mushrooms, and so on
12 cherries (1 choice)	$1/3$ cantaloupe (1 choice)
6 ounces light yogurt (1 choice)	6 ounces light yogurt (1 choice)

As with dinner, you can mix it up by changing your choices. The turkey for the sandwich could be replaced with tuna (with low-fat mayonnaise), ham, lean roast beef, or canned chicken. The chicken in the salad could be replaced with leftover salmon, tuna, boiled eggs, grated reduced-fat cheese, and beans. The pita could be replaced with a slice or two of whole grain bread. Two slices of light wheat bread (two slices of reduced-calorie bread is one choice) could be used to make a whole sandwich for the forty-five-gram carb plan. For the sixty-gram plan half the pita could be replaced with one cup of broth-based soup, which counts as one starch. The lettuce and tomato on the sandwich and the carrots on the side could be replaced with a salad with at least five ingredients. Eight ounces of skim or 1 percent milk could substitute for the light yogurt.

Breakfast: The Most Important Meal of the Day

Breakfasts are typically carb-heavy and fairly low in protein. Adding a protein source often makes this meal more filling. Below are some good breakfast ideas, for both carb budgets (forty-five grams and sixty grams).

Breakfast Planning

45-GRAM CARB BUDGET	60-GRAM CARB BUDGET
1 cup cooked oatmeal (2 choices)	1 whole wheat English muffin (2 choices)
4 ounces of 1 percent milk (1/2 choice)	1 egg, fried in nonstick spray
Half a banana (1/2 choice)	Half a large grapefruit (1 choice)
8 ounces of 1 percent milk (1 choice)	2 teaspoons tub spread for muffin
Coffee or tea	Coffee or tea

There are countless ways to mix it up at breakfast time. The cup of oatmeal can be replaced with 1 1/2 cups of unsweetened dry cereal. The half banana and half serving of milk can be replaced with a whole banana; it's fine to put a dash of milk in your oatmeal (remember, don't sweat the small stuff). One tablespoon of sugar, brown sugar, or honey is one carb choice, so if you want to add a teaspoon or two of sweetener to your oatmeal, just trim back the oatmeal portion a little. The half to whole banana can be replaced with one to two tablespoons of raisins or another dried fruit in your oatmeal or dry cereal. Sprinkle a tablespoon of chopped nuts over your cereal to add a little more protein and fiber. The whole wheat English muffin can be replaced with two slices of whole grain toast, a small (approximately 150-calorie) bagel, two waffles, or two small (four-inch) pancakes. Two egg whites or a half cup of egg substitutes could substitute for the whole egg. In a pinch, a PB&J of one to two tablespoons of peanut butter, a teaspoon or two of 100 percent fruit spread, and two slices of whole wheat bread can be a pretty filling breakfast on the run.

Ideas for Snack Time

By this point you understand the benefits of pairing a carbohydrate with a protein to help make the snack more satisfying and to slow down carb digestion. You use the exchange lists the same way: one carb choice (or maybe two, depending on whether your budget allows for fifteen or thirty grams of carb at a snack) and one protein serving. If you opt for leaner protein choices—or small portions of higher-fat choices—you'll save yourself some calories. These snacks pair one carb choice with one lean protein: six to eight whole grain crackers and one ounce reduced-fat cheese; one apple and one ounce reduced-fat cheese; or half of a six-inch pita with one ounce of turkey (with a touch of mustard or salsa for added flavor).

It's also possible to opt for a higher-fat protein, but it's important to watch your portions to control the calorie content of the snack: six to eight whole wheat crackers with one tablespoon of peanut butter; or one egg and one slice of whole wheat toast (with a small amount of tub spread).

Nuts contain a little protein when eaten in small amounts. Portion control is critical: you don't want heart-healthy nuts to be a major calorie contributor to your diet. For example, mindlessly snacking on a half cup of peanuts will load you down with 425 calories and 36 grams of fat! But a few nuts coupled with a carb can make for a satisfying snack. Here are some great ideas: seventeen grapes plus ten to fifteen peanuts; three-quarters of a cup of unsweetened cereal (or a third of a cup lightly sweetened cereal) and six to eight almonds; or six ounces light yogurt coupled with one tablespoon of chopped walnuts. (See more snack ideas in chapter 10.)

Using Food Labels

You can also use food labels to estimate the carbohydrate content of foods. All the information you need is there. The serving size; the grams of carbohydrate per serving; and the grams of fiber. Remember, if there are more than five grams of fiber, you can subtract half from the total carbs for that food. But the accuracy of your carb count is only as good as you are at judging the portion size. Here's an example of how to estimate an appropriate portion of cereal, for someone aiming for two carb choices worth of cereal (thirty grams of carb) for breakfast:

Fiber Flakes

Serving size: 3/4 cup
Total carbohydrate: 23 grams
Fiber: 5 grams

Because the fiber here is 5 grams or more, you can subtract half the fiber from the total, so there are roughly 20 grams of absorbable fiber in a three-quarter-cup serving. If you divide 20 into 30 you get 1.5 servings, or slightly more than one cup of cereal (0.75 cup × 1.5 = 1.125 cups). If you have an aversion to doing math, don't sweat it. Estimate. Guess. At least you're making an effort to think about the portion. And, again, measure the portion a few times until you become a pretty accurate estimator. It's

> ### A Warning about Food Labels
>
> Don't expect the manufacturer's portion to necessarily be the same as the exchange list. Many store-bought breads, for example, weigh more than one ounce, so they are more than fifteen grams of carb (and more than eighty to ninety calories per slice).

a skill you need to learn to take on the road with you. If you add a glass of milk and a fruit to your portion of cereal (two choices, or 30 grams of carb), you arrive at about 60 grams of carbohydrate for that meal. Aiming for 45 grams? Stick with one serving of cereal, or have half a fruit serving (for example, half of a small banana instead of a whole one) and half of a milk serving (four ounces instead of eight ounces).

A Portion Size Reality Check

All the portions in these examples come from the exchange lists and are designed to help you see what portions we should be eating really look like. When you compare those to what many of us are used to eating, it becomes clear how distorted the modern idea of "normal" portion sizes is. Having said that, by no means do I feel there is a significant difference between eating half-ounce or three-quarters of an ounce of crackers. Or between a four- or five-ounce apple. Those aren't the kinds of portion control errors we're making that have made the United States the most overweight country in the world. The challenges are more on the magnitude of eating portions that are 30 to 50 percent bigger than they should be. One of the hardest things to accept is that there is a certain amount of discomfort that goes along with eating less, mainly because what is often put in front of us—particularly in restaurants and in takeout containers— is excessive. We are required to resist some of the food we're exposed to. And never in the history of the human race have our bodies ever wanted to resist food.

The opposite is true, in fact; for our very survival, humans are strongly hardwired to want to eat whatever we can find. We are now in the unfortunate position, though, of having to resist these instincts. The instincts that genetically served us well are now backfiring, leading to overeating in an environment that requires little of us physically, ultimately resulting in excessive weight gain and chronic health problems. The solution? We must learn to work with our genes, not against them. The more you understand why we do what we do with food, and how absolutely critical regular physical activity is to weight control and good health, the greater our ability to internalize what needs to happen to lose weight and keep it off.

Simple Rules of Carb Counting

The bottom line with carb counting is that it helps you relearn portion sizes of carb-containing foods that have suffered serious portion distortion in your life. Once you've started to orient to more appropriate portions, there are a few simple rules for different food groups that you can apply to healthfully distribute them throughout the day.

Fruit. Whole fruits should be limited to one serving at a time, using the fruit exchange list as a way to estimate a portion. Juice should be limited to no more than four to six ounces a day. One way to include the minimum of two fruits a day is to have one either with breakfast or a midmorning snack and one in the afternoon or evening. According to MyPyramid .gov, the recommended fruit intake for adults is $1^1/_2$ to 2 cups, or the equivalent of about two to four servings of fruit a day.

Milk or yogurt. Eat these food items one serving at a time. If you're having milk with breakfast, have yogurt as a snack in the afternoon. MyPyramid .gov recommends three servings of dairy a day; however, it also counts cheese in the milk group because it is a good source of calcium, whereas the exchange lists count cheese as protein because it contains little to no carbohydrate. For our purposes, aim for two to three servings of milk or yogurt a day, less if you're getting your calcium and protein from other sources. This would be the case with someone who is a vegan (who eats no animal products).

Grains and starchy vegetables. Limit these foods to two servings per meal or to one serving per snack. As per MyPyramid, aim for half of your grains to be whole grains, or for at least three servings of whole grains a day. Because you are following a moderately carbohydrate-restricted diet, you may not be eating quite as many carb servings as is recommended by MyPyramid.

Sweets. Don't just add sweets to your meal or snack—make room for them. Look at the food label if it's available and see how many fifteen-gram carb units a portion of the sweet treat will gobble up. Then look at what else you're planning on eating at that time and eat less of it to make room for a small portion of something sweet. If a food label isn't available, assume that your usual instinct is to eat larger portions than you should, so keep it small.

. . .

The next chapter gets down to one of the greatest challenges for many women: weight loss. Fear of trying to lose weight—and failing—is the bane of many women's existence. Having read this far, perhaps you're already starting to devise a diet approach to get your glucose and insulin levels under control. Managing your insulin response is an important step toward readying your body for weight loss. By now, these changes are probably helping you feel more in control of your hunger.

Mind-Set Intervention: Don't Sweat the Small Stuff!

When you're starting out on the PCOS diet plan, you might begin eating off a smaller plate and aiming for the balanced-plate approach (without counting carbohydrates). Just trading off that extra portion of rice for a serving of vegetables and throwing the rest of your energy at increasing your activity may be all you need—or at least as far as you go in the first few weeks. If you find you really need some clear limits on the amount of carbohydrate you're eating and feel you're not so good at estimating portions, carb counting is likely to be beneficial. But you don't need to jump right into it. Think of learning how to change your diet as climbing a flight of stairs. You start climbing by paying some extra attention to how often you're eating, making more effort to eat your next meal or snack when you start to get hungry—not waiting until you're starving and out of control. The next step may be working toward the balanced plate, but maybe it's not half vegetables initially. A perfectly fine first goal is to consistently add a vegetable to dinner, experimenting with different vegetables you've never tried before, or didn't like earlier in life but might like as an adult. Lasting behavior change comes from creating your own way of doing things, making your own path at your own pace.

Yes, it might take longer than joining a diet program that calls for quick, drastic change, and often resulting in quick weight loss. But did that weight stay off in the long run? Use this as your opportunity to do it *your* way this time, and be flexible about the time frame it takes to achieve your goals. Taking it slow but moving in the right direction beats deciding it's all too hard and doing nothing. Even with slow progress, within a year's time you'll still likely be slimmer, healthier, and more fertile (if that is one of your goals) than you are today.

6

Fighting the Weight War

We've learned about how to manipulate your diet to manage your insulin response and reduce your risk of heart disease and diabetes—two diseases known to be closely tied to polycystic ovary syndrome. Because many women with PCOS are overweight, the ultimate challenge is weight loss, particularly if they want to get pregnant. Losing weight may be a bit more of an uphill battle for women with the condition, but the positive news is that even modest weight loss—5 to 10 percent of your current weight—may be enough to increase fertility and reduce the risk of developing diabetes and other health problems related to PCOS. For example, if you weigh 180 pounds, a weight loss of 5 to 10 percent is 9 to 18 pounds. If you weigh 230 pounds, a weight loss of 5 to 10 percent is roughly 12 to 23 pounds—that kind of weight loss doesn't sound too drastic, does it?

I make this point for a few reasons. I want to make it exceedingly clear that you can lose a very reasonable amount of weight and get significant health results, even if your Body Mass Index (BMI) is still quite a bit above the healthy range. Let's go back to the example of the 230-pound woman, and assume she's five feet, six inches tall. If she loses twenty-three pounds, she will have lost 10 percent of her weight, now weighing in at 207. According to the BMI charts, she'll have a BMI of 33, which still puts her in the obese category, but that's down from a BMI of 37 (when she weighed 230 pounds). Even though you might like to get back into your high school jeans, you can reap significant health benefits from losing modest amounts of weight. Sometimes, at the outset, the journey seems too long. If the very thought of getting your weight into the ideal range—where your BMI is below 25 (which would require our example to get down to 150 pounds)—sounds absolutely overwhelming, that might be enough to discourage you from even trying. An extremely common sentiment is, "If I can't get my weight into that healthy range, why bother?"

In our society we're conditioned to feel like we're supposed to go from overweight to slim and fabulous when we "go on a diet." We tend to rate our success based on how we look (or what the infomercials say we should look like!) versus how much healthier we are. It's not that we don't appreciate the health benefits of weight loss, it's just that it's generally not the main attraction. Given the challenges involved in weight loss, we need to expand our definition of success so we can appreciate the benefits of losing an amount of weight that's reasonable for many people to achieve. This is particularly important if your goal is to become pregnant and reduce your risk of obesity-related pregnancy complications like gestational diabetes. Your likelihood of becoming pregnant and having a healthy pregnancy may improve with a mere 5 to 10 percent weight loss. By all means, think big, but don't lose sight of the value of small successes.

Prone to Being Overweight

Not all women with PCOS are overweight. In fact, I've had several women with PCOS in my practice who were quite thin yet still don't ovulate and experienced some (although generally milder) symptoms of elevated androgens. But the fact is that more women with PCOS are overweight than aren't, and this condition carries with it some special challenges. The reasons for higher rates of obesity when you have PCOS are likely multifactorial, having to do with a combined effect of genetic predisposition, hormonal imbalances that can affect your appetite and ability to feel full, and the usual obesogenic influences (poor diet and reduced activity) we're all subjected to.

Fluctuations in insulin levels can aggravate hunger and lead to cravings for carbohydrates in many people. Research suggests that women with PCOS may have some deviation from normal of the hunger and satiety hormones ghrelin and leptin. *Ghrelin* is the hormone that makes us feel hungry, and *leptin* is the hormone that helps us feel full. Women with PCOS may maintain higher ghrelin levels after eating, helping to explain why many women with PCOS report difficulty feeling full.[1] There also appears to be a connection between leptin and insulin resistance, although how this relates to PCOS is still under investigation.[2] An additional challenge may be that women with the syndrome, particularly those who test positive for insulin resistance on a glucose tolerance test, may have a slower metabolic rate, making them more prone to weight gain.[3] Not to be ignored is the fact that having PCOS is downright stressful, which in and of itself may lead these women to seek solace in food!

Why Weight Loss Helps

Scientists have established that weight gain in women both with and without PCOS aggravates insulin resistance (although women with the condition tend to be more insulin resistant when compared with women of the same age and BMI without PCOS). The combined effects of genetic predisposition and an obesogenic environment are likely responsible for the higher rates of obesity seen in women with PCOS.[4] That means you may have a genetic predisposition to obesity because you have the syndrome, so when your genetics interface with modern society's norm of eating too much and exercising too little, it's like pouring lighter fluid on the fire of PCOS. Simply put, you have the genes for PCOS, so you start to gain weight. The weight gain aggravates the underlying hormone imbalances associated with PCOS (insulin resistance, hyperandrogenism), you begin to experience more hunger from the insulin resistance, you gain weight more easily, and you experience more symptoms of PCOS.

We also know that abdominal obesity (the apple shape) is more prevalent in women with PCOS, affecting more than half of women with the condition.[5] Because belly fat is associated with both elevated insulin levels and androgens, this sets the stage for a vicious cycle, where having belly fat makes you more insulin resistant, which increases androgen production, which encourages more depositing of fat in the abdomen. And so on, and so on, and so on. You may feel stuck in your attempts to lose weight because the condition itself is undermining your efforts. However, we know that losing just some of that belly fat improves fertility and lowers the risk of developing diabetes. This is why it's so important to get the insulin resistance under control. It can help level the playing field and make it easier to lose weight.

Research also supports that weight loss in women with PCOS helps reduce circulating androgens, raises sex hormone binding globulin (which binds androgens, making them less active), enhances insulin sensitivity, and improves ovulation and fertility. Even modest amounts of weight loss can improve response to fertility treatments like IUI (intrauterine insemination) and IVF (in vitro fertilization).[6] A study from the University of Milan in Italy took thirty-three overweight women with PCOS who were not ovulating (six) or ovulated irregularly (twenty-seven). After following a calorie-restricted diet and being advised to do some aerobic exercise throughout the week (a minimum of once or twice per week), the improvements in their fertility were dramatic.

- Twenty-five of the thirty-three women lost at least 5 percent of their body weight; 11 percent of the women lost 10 percent of their body weight.
- Waist circumference, BMI, and fat mass were significantly reduced after weight loss of 5 percent or more.
- The women's ovarian size and microfollicule number was reduced significantly.
- Of the women with irregular periods, eighteen resumed regular cycles and fifteen spontaneously ovulated.
- Ten spontaneous pregnancies occurred in the women who lost at least 5 percent of their body weight.[7]

Body Mass Index: Evaluating Your Weight

When figuring out your health goals, it makes sense to start by evaluating your weight first. That used to involve looking at a height-weight chart at the doctor's office based on whether you were small-, medium-, or large-framed. There's a new chart in town: the Body Mass Index. BMI is also calculated using a person's height and weight and is considered a reliable indicator of body fatness. It does not measure body fat directly, but research has shown that BMI correlates to direct measures of body fat, such as underwater weighing, which is considered the gold standard of body composition measurement. BMI is used as a way to determine at what weight you may begin to experience an increase in health problems. It is figured using a complex calculation (weight in kilograms divided by height in meters squared), but anyone with Internet access can bypass the math by using an online BMI calculator.[8] You can also use the BMI chart below. Find your height and weight and see where your BMI shakes out.

Body Mass Index Table

	Normal						Overweight					Obese										Extreme Obesity							
BMI	19	20	21	22	23	24	25	26	27	28	29	30	31	32	33	34	35	36	37	38	39	40	41	42	43	44	45	46	47
Height (inches)											Body Weight (pounds)																		
58	91	96	100	105	110	115	119	124	129	134	138	143	148	153	158	162	167	172	177	181	186	191	196	201	205	210	215	220	224
59	94	99	104	109	114	119	124	128	133	138	143	148	153	158	163	168	173	178	183	188	193	198	203	208	212	217	222	227	232
60	97	102	107	112	118	123	128	133	138	143	148	153	158	163	168	174	179	184	189	194	199	204	209	215	220	225	230	235	240
61	100	106	111	116	122	127	132	137	143	148	153	158	164	169	174	180	185	190	195	201	206	211	217	222	227	232	238	243	248
62	104	109	115	120	126	131	136	142	147	153	158	164	169	175	180	186	191	196	202	207	213	218	224	229	235	240	246	251	256
63	107	113	118	124	130	135	141	146	152	158	163	169	175	180	186	191	197	203	208	214	220	225	231	237	242	248	254	259	265
64	110	116	122	128	134	140	145	151	157	163	169	174	180	186	192	197	204	209	215	221	227	232	238	244	250	256	262	267	273
65	114	120	126	132	138	144	150	156	162	168	174	180	186	192	198	204	210	216	222	228	234	240	246	252	258	264	270	276	282
66	118	124	130	136	142	148	155	161	167	173	179	186	192	198	204	210	216	223	229	235	241	247	253	260	266	272	278	284	291
67	121	127	134	140	146	153	159	166	172	178	185	191	198	204	211	217	223	230	236	242	249	255	261	268	274	280	287	293	299
68	125	131	138	144	151	158	164	171	177	184	190	197	203	210	216	223	230	236	243	249	256	262	269	276	282	289	295	302	308
69	128	135	142	149	155	162	169	176	182	189	196	203	209	216	223	230	236	243	250	257	263	270	277	284	291	297	304	311	318
70	132	139	146	153	160	167	174	181	188	195	202	209	216	222	229	236	243	250	257	264	271	278	285	292	299	306	313	320	327
71	136	143	150	157	165	172	179	186	193	200	208	215	222	229	236	243	250	257	265	272	279	286	293	301	308	315	322	329	338
72	140	147	154	162	169	177	184	191	199	206	213	221	228	235	242	250	258	265	272	279	287	294	302	309	316	324	331	338	346
73	144	151	159	166	174	182	189	197	204	212	219	227	235	242	250	257	265	272	280	288	295	302	310	318	325	333	340	348	355

Once you know your BMI, you can determine whether you're already at a healthy weight or are considered "overweight," or "obese," or "extremely obese." Keep in mind that these BMI interpretations are designed for people over age twenty. For children and teens, you can find appropriate calculators online.[9] Although the number is calculated the same way, the interpretation of BMI for growing children is different, as it needs to be evaluated on a percentile growth curve that compares the child to other children of the same age and sex.

Body Mass Index and Weight Status

BMI	WEIGHT STATUS
Less than 18.5	Underweight
18.5–24.9	Normal
25–29.9	Overweight
30 and above	Obese

However, there are some limitations with the BMI system. Because BMI is calculated using weight that includes both lean and fat mass, a small percentage of people may fall into the "overweight" range because they have excess muscle. This might be the case with a competitive athlete, but that would be limited to some drifting into the "overweight" range. Most people with a BMI above 30 will have excess body fatness. The other limitation of BMI is that it's only *one* indicator of overall health—the others being diet, activity level, and family and health history.

Thinking about "Health" versus "Pounds"

The BMI ranges are based on the relationship between body weight and disease and death. Overweight and obese individuals are at increased risk for many health problems, including hypertension, high LDL cholesterol, low HDL cholesterol, high levels of triglycerides in your blood, type 2 diabetes, heart disease, stroke, gallbladder problems, arthritis, sleep apnea, respiratory problems, and some cancers (endometrial, breast, colon, and possibly others). Before you get too overwhelmed by your BMI number as it correlates with this list of health consequences, let me say it again: Just because you can't imagine getting your BMI down to the below-25 range does not mean weight loss isn't worth it. Even if you don't get close to a BMI of 25, losing just enough weight to avoid getting diabetes is completely worth it. Ask anyone with diabetes whether they'd rather invest their time working on diet and lifestyle change to avoid getting diabetes versus expending energy learning how to balance diet, activity, and medications to control diabetes once they have it. The majority of people would wish they hadn't waited to make changes. Work on it now or work on it later—in both situations diet and activity habits have to change.

Since the mid-1950s, the general approach to losing weight in the United States has been "to go on a diet." There have been countless ones to choose from over the years, with most diets involving a sudden, dramatic change in what you eat. Some diets have recommended eliminating whole food groups (fat, carbs, white flour, junk food). Other diet plans offer to make it easy by providing you with packaged food so you don't have to spend much time thinking about what you're going to eat. Many require you to cut your calories way back, maybe as low as a thousand calories a day. Some diets are even lower in calories, usually as part of a medically supervised diet that has you drink protein-packed milkshakes a few times a day. Regardless of the specific approach, what most fad diets have had in common is radical dietary change, with the unspoken promise that if you just "stick to the rules," you'll lose a bunch of weight. This translates into: "If I just behave myself and stop acting so weak around food, I'll be able to lose weight." That kind of thinking puts responsibility for whether you succeed on the diet or not squarely on your shoulders—if you lost weight, you were virtuous and good; if you didn't, you were weak and untrustworthy around food.

Most diets like this are doomed to fail because they threaten your body's internal instincts geared toward self-preservation; they don't focus enough on providing skills to make permanent change. Any dietary changes that cut your calories back will result in weight loss. We may know that what we're doing to lose weight we can't possibly maintain for the long haul, or that we shouldn't lose the weight that way because it's not healthy, but somehow we hold out hope that this "new diet" will be the one that doesn't result in us regaining the weight. But think about it: If at the end of a "diet" that was not sustainable you drift back to the diet and lifestyle habits that got you into trouble in the first place, why wouldn't you get the same result?

Deep down we know this, but long-term change is so challenging that we really don't want to believe it. Stop thinking about "dieting" and start framing the weight-loss issue as something that should happen as a result of focusing on developing healthier habits. The things that you would do to reduce your risk of developing diabetes, control your blood pressure, lower your risk of cancer, and in general help yourself feel physically and mentally better in your body every day are the same things that should result in weight loss. It is never a bad thing to think about health versus pounds. I've had many clients who lose weight for the first time in a long time, after achieving a better understanding of what it takes to control insulin resistance. With this other significant focus, they've been able to avoid the psychological baggage that often comes along with "dieting."

Mind-Set Intervention: Staying in the Game!

The whole concept of "dieting" tends to psychologically bring out the worst in us. No one can be meaner or less forgiving of ourselves than us. Ever had these thoughts when contemplating going on a weight-loss diet? *I can't do this. I've tried this so many times before and failed. Why bother? My body is just incapable of weight loss. I'm addicted to food and no diet is going to fix that. I have no self-control. I always seem to drift back to this place that gets me into trouble. I'm so uncoordinated. Exercise is so uncomfortable for me.*

This is just the tip of the iceberg of some of the negative self-talk I've heard expressed over the years by people who are unhappy with their weight. It's easy to see how one could focus on past failures. Trying so hard at something only to be unsuccessful in the long term hurts! But you have two choices: (1) keep doing what you're doing and become increasingly unhappy about the state of your health or quality of life, or (2) start chipping away at it in a positive direction. The beauty of the PCOS diet plan is that it can help you achieve your goals from a whole new angle, by taking you down a road you've never traveled before. You're changing behaviors to help regulate your hormones and overall health using positive steps to nudge out the unhealthy habits. Changes should be made gradually, in a step-by-step manner, focusing on one or two goals at a time. This is very different from "dieting."

Being a Successful Loser

In 1994, Dr. Rena Wing of Brown University and Dr. James Hill of the University of Colorado founded the National Weight Control Registry (NWCR) to help identify a large sample of people who had lost weight and successfully kept it off long term.[10] The NWCR recruits participants who are eighteen years or older, have maintained a weight loss of at least thirty pounds, and kept it off for at least one year. Registry members provide information yearly via questionnaires on eating habits, activity patterns, and weight-control strategies. To date there are more than six thousand participants in the NWCR, and a new Teenage NWCR is in the works.

Who *are* these successful losers? Demographically, the National Weight Control Registry participants share a lot in common: 95 percent of them are Caucasian, 77 percent are female, 82 percent are college educated, 64 percent are married. Efforts are currently under way to diversify the gender, ethnic, and socioeconomic status of the group. The average BMI before starting to lose weight is 36.7, well into the "obese" range. Upon entry to the NWCR, the average member had lost seventy-four pounds (with a range from thirty to three hundred pounds!), and reduced their BMI to 25.2 (almost in the "normal" range). About 44 percent of them lost weight on their own; 55.4 percent participated in group programs (such as Weight Watchers and Overeaters Anonymous) or in individual counseling with a therapist or dietitian.

Although many weight-loss programs are able to consistently produce weight losses of 7 to 10 percent of initial body weight within six to twelve months, many people who lose weight regain it within a relatively short period of time. Why is it so difficult to lose weight and keep it off? Although we don't have all the answers to this question, we know a few factors play a role in maintaining weight loss. Physiological changes that occur during weight loss, such as a decline in metabolic rate and changes in thyroid and hunger hormone activity, can make it tougher to feel satisfied and easier to eat more than we need. Psychological and behavioral changes—boredom with food choices, decreased motivation over time once the novelty of looser clothing and better health wears off—can also be tough to sustain. What is clear is that to lose weight and keep it off you need to strive for permanent, sustainable change. Finding ongoing support for that from friends, family, health-care providers, and group support is critical.

Common Strategies of NWCR Participants

The vast majority of NWCR participants (89 percent) used both diet and physical activity to lose weight. Just 10 percent changed only their diet, and 1 percent changed only their level of activity. Less common strategies employed to lose weight were using liquid meal replacements (13.8 percent), weight-loss medications (6.2 percent), and surgery (2.4 percent). As for dietary changes, the three most common weight-loss techniques employed were (1) limiting intake of foods associated with weight gain, like sweets and fatty items, including desserts; (2) decreasing portion sizes of all foods; and (3) counting calories (about 50 percent of NWCR participants report counting calories or fat grams).

For physical activity, 92 percent of participants exercise at home, with walking and aerobic dancing more common in women and competitive sports and weightlifting more common in men. A large group (about 40 percent) use the buddy system by exercising with a friend, and about 31 percent exercise as part of a group. Equally impressive are the participants' reported quality-of-life scores after losing the weight and maintaining the loss:

- Almost all participants (95.3 percent) reported improvements in quality of life (both physical and psychological).
- Almost all (92.4 percent) experienced improved energy and mobility, making physical activity more possible.
- Mood improved as well, with 91.4 percent reporting decreases in symptoms of depression.

This last point is particularly important. Studies show that regain after weight loss is significantly more common in people who feel more depressed (and who are prone to uncontrolled eating, often in response to stress).

Successful Strategies for Maintenance

Despite some variation in approaches to weight loss, when it comes to maintenance of that loss, there are many common strategies among the "losers." In terms of what they ate, though not perfect, successful losers seem a bit better than the average American at managing their eating according to health experts' recommendations.[11] The following statistics are only averages, so there is definitely a range of intake of carbohydrates, protein, and fat among the NWCR participants. Most importantly, successful losers report being constantly vigilant about what they eat. Calorie intake is maintained at a fairly low level—on average about fourteen hundred calories. The NWCR founders speculate that these low numbers may reflect the fact that many of the participants reported they were still trying to lose weight. Keep in mind that studies show that people, particularly those who are overweight, are notorious for underreporting food intake, so a reported intake of fourteen hundred calories may actually be higher.

Average fat intake is reported to be quite low, averaging about 24 percent of calories (definitely a low-fat diet), or about 45 grams a day. More recent participants report a fat intake of about 29 percent, likely reflecting the recent popularity of low-carb diets. Carb intake has declined over the past few years but still averages out at about 53 percent of calories, or 182 grams a day. Protein intake is about 19 percent of calories, or about 64 grams per day. Registry participants eat their veggies, an average of four servings a day, and eat more fiber from fruits, vegetables, and beans than from grains. Breakfast is a must among 78 percent of NWCR participants, supporting reams of research tying breakfast intake with weight loss (and less eating at night!). Most prepare their meals at home and rarely eat fast food (less than once a week on average). Counter to the common American trend of dining out, registry participants apparently recognize the challenges, eating outside the home only three times a week.

Eating patterns matter as well. The average NWCR member eats about five times a day, suggesting they make efforts to stay ahead of their hunger to avoid overeating. They also tend to be consistent in their eating, trying to maintain calorie control on the weekends and around the holidays—a habit that counters the approach of dieting during the week and letting loose on the weekends. More than 75 percent weigh themselves more than once a week. Participants find that monitoring their weight helps guide their diet and physical activity choices and allows them to get right on any regain when it's only a pound or two. Think about it: if you don't weigh yourself, how can you know if you're drifting? Weighing also tells you when things are going well—hard to appreciate if you tend to associate weighing with delivering only bad news.

For successful maintenance, exercise plays a major role. About 76 percent walk, 20 percent lift weights, and 20 percent cycle, for an average of about sixty minutes a day. (These are moderate-intensity activities. According to government guidelines, sixty minutes of moderate activity can be replaced with thirty minutes of intense activity, like running or high-intensity aerobics). Time spent on physical activity likely comes at the cost of "screen time"—the average registry member watches only six to ten hours of TV, compared with twenty-eight hours a week for the average American.

What's clear from NWCR member feedback is that they spend a substantial amount of time and energy on these strategies and strive to be as consistent as possible. When they begin to regain weight, it is most likely to happen in the early stages of maintenance and is most often associated with drifting from these strategies. On the positive side members report that it gets easier to maintain weight loss over time. Once they've maintained a weight loss for two to five years, their chances of long-term success increase greatly.

Lessons from Successful Losers

Losing weight and keeping it off is certainly challenging, but not impossible. Losing weight positively affects every physical and emotional quality-of-life indicator. It requires some support from another person (a coach, counselor, or exercise buddy) or a group. Preliminary research suggests that face-to-face support is best, but some people find what they need from an online source, like a weight-loss program website, a chat room, or a blog. Maintaining your weight loss can be even more challenging, as it requires swimming upstream against social norms. Eating out too often makes it hard to control calorie intake. The portion distortion we're exposed to in restaurants makes it hard to remember what a "normal" size portion is. Too much time spent on the computer or watching TV can monopolize time that could otherwise be spent getting some physical activity.

The ultimate ambition of the NWCR is to teach aspiring "losers" the skills that may help them succeed. The registry founder's STOP Regain study demonstrated this possibility by recruiting 314 people who had lost at least 10 percent of their initial body weight over the previous two years (most had lost almost 20 percent of their initial weight) and teaching them the habits of the NWCR participants. These "lessons" were shared in weekly meetings for a month, followed by monthly meetings for eighteen months total. The results? Compared to a group that had no intervention, the STOP Regain program participants regained significantly less weight.[12] It comes down to support and choices.

The NWCR itself gleans limited information about its members' attitudes, but other studies have looked at the emotional aspects at play in those who've achieved lasting weight loss. Registered dietitian Anne M. Fletcher, author of *Thin for Life: Ten Keys to Success from People Who Have Lost Weight and Kept It Off*, which captures the strategies of more than two hundred adults who have maintained weight loss, says "These 'masters' of former weight problems recognize that there's no such thing as perfection when it comes to weight control. When they 'slip'—for instance, eat in a way they hadn't intended or miss a day of exercise—they don't berate themselves. Instead, they prevent such lapses from becoming full-blown relapses by picking up right where they left off." One woman interviewed by Fletcher said that when she doesn't handle a food situation the way she would have liked, she doesn't fixate on it or berate herself. Instead, "I get it in perspective: that one candy bar won't make me twenty pounds overweight. I look at the big picture. I remind myself that there are a multitude of things I do in a day, in a week, like eating breakfast, exercising, and drinking water, that help me maintain my weight. That one candy bar is a drop in the bucket."[13]

Masters of weight control also seem to be resilient and able to learn from past experiences. Fletcher found that it's not uncommon for those who ultimately succeed at lasting weight loss to have lost weight and regained it numerous times in the past. Nearly eight out of ten of the weight maintainers Fletcher interviewed had tried to lose weight at least three or four times before they finally succeeded. "Rather than let these attempts serve as cruel reminders of failure," Fletcher advises, "it's more useful to view past dieting efforts as learning opportunities, to identify what did and didn't work for you in the past." One woman who had lost and kept off thirty-five pounds for ten years said, "If you hate fish, don't eat it just to lose weight." Fletcher suggests making two lists, one of strategies that have worked for you in past dieting attempts (for example, getting up to eat breakfast or walking the dog after work) and a second list of strategies that have not worked (such as eating grapefruit with every meal or getting up to go swimming at 5 a.m.). As you get serious about managing your weight again in a healthy way, employ only those strategies that truly have worked in the past.

Incorporating NWCR Strategies into the PCOS Diet Plan

Let's compare the recommendations from the PCOS diet plan with the successful NWCR strategies. Despite the need for some fine-tuning because the PCOS diet plan is specific to managing insulin resistance, there is quite a bit of overlap.

Comparing Recommendations:
The PCOS Diet Plan and NWCR Strategies

PCOS DIET PLAN	NWCR STRATEGIES
Spread carbs out over three meals and two to three snacks per day.	Eat an average of four to five times per day.
Cover half your plate with vegetables.	Eat four or more servings of vegetables daily.
Start the day with a protein-containing breakfast.	Eat breakfast daily.
Eat proactively to stay ahead of hunger.	Be continuously vigilant about portions and control portion sizes.
Budget out time each week to shop and plan meals to control choices.	Prepare most of your own meals.
Budget out time for daily activity to help manage your insulin resistance.	Be moderately active for sixty minutes daily.
Eat carbohydrates in moderation; don't overrestrict.	Eat carbohydrates in moderation; don't overrestrict.
Limit your fat intake to help control calories.	Follow a low-fat diet.
Eat protein in moderation—enough to help you feel full but not so much that you're getting too many calories.	Eat protein in moderation.
Control your food environment to limit temptations.	Limit eating out to three times weekly.
Focus on the positive; learn and move on from lapses.	Lapses are opportunities to learn, not evidence of weakness or failure.

As you can see, there isn't one diet and lifestyle strategy for managing PCOS and another one for weight loss. They both accomplish the same thing! If weight loss is not your goal, you may need to increase lean protein and healthy fat intake slightly to help fill the void left by trimming carbohydrates. Or you may need to add an extra snack. In any case, the goal of the PCOS diet plan is to kill multiple birds with one stone (manage insulin resistance, reduce the risk for diabetes and heart disease, lose weight if necessary, enhance fertility)—without compromising the overall quality of the diet.

Figuring out Protein Intake

One potential difference between the PCOS diet plan and the recommendations from the NWCR is the protein intake. Whereas the NWCR folks average about 19 percent of their calories from protein, with PCOS you may need to eat a little more. According to the Dietary Guidelines for Americans, protein intake can healthfully provide anywhere from 10 to 35 percent of daily calories. In the PCOS diet plan protein intake averages about 21 to 22 percent of daily calories—still well within the healthy range. The key is to choose lean choices so your protein foods don't come packaged with a lot of fat.

Overall, when it comes to weight loss, research is mixed on whether eating more or less of any one nutrient (carbohydrate, protein, or fat) is more effective than any other. One recent study from the Brigham and Women's Hospital in Boston of more than eight hundred people trying to lose weight tested four different diets. Each provided a different amount of calories from carbohydrate, protein, and fat. The fat ranged from 20 to 40 percent of calories, protein from 15 to 25 percent of calories, and carbohydrate from 35 to 65 percent of calories. All groups were offered individual and group support for two years. The results? All groups lost about the same amount of weight. All groups also experienced improvements in their blood lipid and insulin levels. Not surprisingly, attending the group sessions was strongly associated with weight loss.[14]

The take-home message is that cutting calories is what counts most, and there are many means of achieving that. What's unique about managing PCOS is the two-pronged goal: weight loss and managing insulin response. Clearly, losing weight helps manage the insulin response, but managing the insulin response can also make weight loss easier. Because eating less carbohydrate at one sitting (particularly when it's paired with protein and a little healthy fat) will mute the demand for insulin, our goal is to include enough protein to help make eating less carbohydrate easier. From a physiological standpoint there are several reasons why eating a bit more protein may help with weight loss:

- Protein generally increases fullness to a greater extent than carbohydrate or fat, and so may help you eat fewer calories at a meal or snack.
- Higher-protein diets are associated with increased thermogenesis, meaning that your body burns more calories processing it, which in turn promotes fullness.
- For some people, eating more protein may help them retain more muscle while they're losing weight.[15]

Research backs up this more-protein approach. One study of women from the University of Illinois at Urbana-Champaign compared a higher-carbohydrate diet (68 grams of protein a day) versus a higher-protein diet (125 grams of protein a day). After ten weeks the women lost about the same amount of weight, but the women in the higher-protein group had a significantly higher loss of body fat. The women with the higher-carbohydrate intake had higher insulin responses to meals and more post-meal hypoglycemia (which causes hunger), whereas the women in the higher-protein group reported greater satiety (fullness) after meals and significant reductions in unhealthy blood triglyceride levels.[16] One small study in 2009 sought to test this out in women with PCOS by cutting calories in two groups of women and then adding back 240 calories in the form of either a protein supplement or simple sugar supplement. At the end of the study the protein-supplemented women lost more weight and body fat and had greater improvements in blood cholesterol levels.[17] It bears repeating, however, that this research doesn't support the use of a very low-carb, very high-protein diet for weight loss. We're talking balance here: trimming out most processed carbs in favor of whole grains, beans, fruits, and vegetables, and replacing some of those calories with a bit more lean protein.

Helpful Strategies for Diet and Lifestyle Change

In addition to the strategies recommended by the NWCR, many others are helpful for trying to lose weight. These recommendations are based more on behavior than food. Note the strategies below that might be helpful to you:

Strategy #1: Learn How Your Body Works— It's Not the Enemy!

Before you start thinking you're doomed to a life of squirreling away calories, understand this: It's not that your body won't give up fat, you just don't want to cut your calorie intake so drastically that your body thinks there's a food shortage coming on. That means weeding out a few calories here and there by cutting back your portions, reducing your fat intake, opting for calorie-free beverages, and eating on a regular basis throughout the day to avoid extreme hunger. This way you're doing your best to tell your body that food is still out there without shocking it into calorie-conserving defense mode. If your body thinks the food supply is drying up, it might take action to conserve its calorie burning to preserve what it has.

If your body thinks you've gone too long without food, it's going to stimulate you to stock up when you finally get some. After all, if you were a cave woman and you hadn't eaten in a while and then killed an antelope, are you going to eat like you're at a tea party? Of course not! You're likely to eat fast and furious, beyond fullness, in preparation for the reality that

Coping with Lapses

Some things that can veer us off course can be wonderful, unavoidable events in our lives. I don't expect someone to eat perfectly on her honeymoon or in the weeks after having a baby. But there are some common bumps that are worth developing some strategies for. There are many things you can do to help steer clear of the ditch the next time you lapse. When you overate at a restaurant, maybe you were overhungry when you got there. Next time try to have a carb-protein snack midafternoon and a fruit on the way to the restaurant. It might make it easier to order a healthier option. Also, be careful with whom you dine. Eating out with overeaters may make it feel okay to step out of your healthy habits. If you grabbed takeout on the way home from work, maybe it was because you skipped your usual Sunday trip to the supermarket. Next time schedule it into your calendar to make sure you don't forget.

If you skipped your trip to the gym on the way home from the office because you forgot your gym clothes, try packing a back-up gym bag with an old pair of sneakers, shorts, and a T-shirt that you can leave in your trunk. If you ended up grabbing a snack from the work vending machine, remind yourself how important it is to bring a snack from home. And do it tonight before you go to bed! If you skipped breakfast because you were running late and, as a result, overindulged at lunch, set your clock a few minutes earlier so you have more time in the morning to fit it in. Eating breakfast—or skipping it—tends to set the eating tone for the day: you're either eating proactively to stay ahead of your hunger or reactively in response to being overhungry.

If you found yourself at dinnertime not having eaten any plant foods throughout the day, make a run to the farmers' market or grocery store and be sure to pack fruits and vegetables with your lunch and snacks. Store them where you can see them. Studies show that we're more likely to eat what's in front of us, so keep that apple or banana right on your desk at work and a fruit bowl on the kitchen counter. If you ended up eating Oreos in front of the TV after dinner, be realistic with yourself: don't bring them into the house in the first place! Making treats less accessible removes the impulse to snack on nutrient-poor, high-sugar foods. Instead, try a sugar-free Jell-O, a cup of herbal tea, or a piece of gum while you work on deconditioning yourself from eating in front of the TV.

you may not eat again for a long time. When does this most often happen? At night, of course! The day's been crazy, and there was little time to eat. But once you get home, watch out! Your primitive cave girl instinct kicks in, triggering binge eating. We see this as more evidence of our weakness around food, but your body thinks it's doing you a favor after a long day of being deprived of food.

The solution is to not let yourself get too hungry. Be sure to eat a satisfying breakfast, a filling lunch that includes protein and plant foods, a satiating carbohydrate-protein snack when your hunger starts to kick in midafternoon, and a dinner early enough in the evening that you're not ravenous when you sit down. Think of rating your hunger on a scale of one to ten (one being "not hungry" and ten being "starved") Your best bet is to eat your next meal when your hunger is a five or six. If you wait until it's an eight or a ten, you'll most likely overreact and overeat when you finally get around food. The lesson here is to be a good cave woman and start thinking of eating as a *positive* thing. Going out of your way to eat may actually help you lose weight by helping your body feel it's okay to burn calories and help you stay ahead of your hunger. Make time for a good breakfast. Digesting and processing food uses up about 10 percent of all the calories we burn, so pumping up your metabolic rate with breakfast, then continuing to throw wood on the fire of your metabolism throughout the day (by eating every four hours or so) is actually a great way to stoke your metabolic rate, send your body a positive message about the food supply, and meet your nutrient needs.

Strategy #2: Adjust Your Attitude to Avoid "I'm a Failure" Syndrome

According to NWCR founder Dr. Rena Wing, successful losers are encouraged to view lapses as opportunities to learn, not evidence of weakness or failure. I can't emphasize enough the importance of this. People who lose weight and keep it off don't hope there won't be any bumps in the road to losing weight. Rather, they accept there will be many obstacles along the way, and they try to develop strategies to manage them. One behavior often present in those who lose weight and regain it is how they handle veering off track from their plan. For example, they go out and overeat with friends, take a vacation, have a baby, get married, or someone dies—really any life event, positive or negative, that can make it hard to keep strictly to a program. But the ones who regain the weight frequently allow themselves to skid into the ditch and stay there. There's a tendency to interpret these situations as personal failings, followed by a lot of negative self-talk about weaknesses. The temptation to focus on past failures is great. Such negative thinking puts many people at very high risk of a "what the heck, why bother" reaction.

A much more productive response, however, is to analyze the situation to see if the lapse could have been abbreviated or avoided. Reflect on what happened, why it happened, determine whether it was avoidable, and whether there's a strategy that could help you deal with it should that situation arise again. It's the old cowboy strategy: Pick yourself up, dust yourself off, and get back in the saddle. What else *can* you do? Languishing in negative thinking and reverting back to old habits is going to land you back at square one. Why not just regroup and then get back in the game?

Strategy #3: Keep a Food Journal

Maintaining a food journal is one of the few things that many studies have shown help people keep healthy eating on their radar. Before you groan about it, this can be really easy. Buy a colorful notebook or journal that will get your attention. Some people keep a food log online (see the Resources at the back of the book for some ideas) or even on their cell phone. Throughout the day, you'll record the time, food or beverage consumed, and the amount. Trying to record after the fact will likely result in lost benefit (you may be unlikely to recall every little detail of what you've consumed). It may help to add a "hunger" column to your journal, where you record your hunger on that one-to-ten scale. These notes may remind you to eat when your hunger is a five or six.

Keeping track of what you eat can help in a variety of ways. Initially, it's like conducting an audit of what you're really eating and drinking throughout the day. People do audits at work all the time to figure out where the problem areas are so they can identify solutions. Same thing here: Writing it all down helps you figure out what's working well and what needs to change. Beyond the initial audit, keeping a food journal is a way to keep your goals of diet and behavior change in front of your face.

Every time you pull out your notebook or journal, it's a reminder of what you're trying to accomplish. (See a sample food journal on page 228.)

Strategy #4: Don't Eat Too Much at Night

It's long been known that night-shift workers and those with "night-eating syndrome" (an eating disorder where people wake and eat at night) are prone to being overweight. In my experience people who struggle with their weight often eat too little during the day and too much at night. A similar pattern emerges where food intake tends to escalate as the day goes on. They may or may not eat breakfast or lunch, then find themselves starving by late afternoon and respond to it by diving into the vending machine or business meeting leftovers. They may then come home after work and eat a large dinner and often snack again later in the evening. The end result, of course, is these folks end up eating the bulk of their calories for the day at a time when their body is preparing to go into hibernation mode during sleep.

If this sounds like you, it's no wonder you might not be hungry for breakfast! The good news is that these same people often immediately start to lose weight once they switch to three meals and a snack or two during the day. Simply spreading out their food throughout the day either stimulates their body to let go of some reserves or helps them curb the quantity of their food intake. In either case the effect is positive.

Strategy #5: Accept That There's Some Discomfort Involved

Let's face it. We're hardwired to desire food, wherever and whenever we can get it, and in our society we're overexposed to it. Most of us also have more things on our to-do list than we can possibly accomplish in a day, making exercise seem like one more demand on our time. But what's wrong with this picture is not our bodies, it's our culture. Food is over-available, and very little about modern life demands much of us physically. This unfortunately leaves us in a position where we have to intentionally resist the temptations of our food environment and intentionally insert time for activity.

If we designed a pie chart of all the things that make our life unique, there would be family, friends, work, hobbies, pets, and other important things people work into their lives. To be healthy in this culture, you also need to carve out a piece of the pie to devote to self-care: buying healthy food, preparing and eating it; budgeting in time for physical activity; getting at least seven hours of sleep a night (the amount researchers believe we need for good health); and managing our stress (much of which might be taken care of by regular exercise).

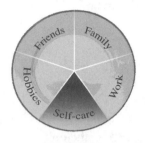

Making this happen isn't easy, but neither is any major accomplishment in life. Healthy eating requires some time and attention so you have decent food in front of you when you sit down to eat a meal or snack. We could all use a personal chef, but unless that's in your budget it's up to you to manage your food environment. Populate your inner food world—think of it as the spaces you move through throughout the day—with things you want to be eating. Make those things you know you should limit a stretch. If fruits, vegetables, whole grains, low-fat dairy, and lean protein is closest at hand, that's what you're most likely to default to. For those of you living with a partner, it's time for a little healthy selfishness! The other people in your house may not be ready to make change, but that doesn't mean you need to make your job harder by catering to different tastes. Healthy eating trumps junk food. Anything you do to improve the food environment at home almost always trickles down to others living there, which is especially important if you have children. Do it for yourself and others will reap the benefits too!

Strategy #6: Focus on the Positive

Healthy eating is more about going out of your way to get good foods into your body than taking foods away. If you add enough foods that are nutritious and filling, there will be less room for the less desirable stuff. Taking a positive approach involves accepting that the process takes time—it's not something that can magically be done quickly. Remember the advice of Dr. Woods from Tufts University's School on Nutrition that significant dietary change results from traveling through a multistep process. Most people get going on steps one and two—they cut out some junk and start to make substitutions—but they never really follow through to step three:

being consistent. Some of that is a result of the frustration with not getting fast results when you opt for a gradual process. But the positive approach is about accepting that you're in it for the long haul. This is a multisemester class, not a crash course. Studies show that slower weight loss is more likely to be permanent.

Strategy #7: Make Losing Weight a Priority

The time to make these important changes happen will not simply fall into your lap, I assure you. It's funny, we can always find time to surf the Internet or watch TV. But taking a long brisk walk, getting out to the farmers' market for fresh vegetables, or logging daily intake in your food journal? You may be having trouble squeezing in those responsibilities. Maybe your new priority is not to watch TV or get online until you've taken care of these important tasks. You also may need to push back on all the people and other things that make demands on your time. Find the time, make it a priority. This is your health we're talking about.

Strategy #8: Manage Your Mind-Set and Your Expectations

No doubt, making these diet and lifestyle changes can be difficult, especially if you have years of dieting under your belt. It can be hard to shake off the negative thinking and overly ambitious expectations. Try ascribing to a few basic assumptions to help you steer around some of the sticking points of the past:

- You can't change the past, but you can learn from it.
- Change is tough. Go easy on yourself. So what if it takes longer? Slowly dipping into the things you find challenging a little at a time may feel less threatening than jumping in with both barrels drawn!
- Focus on getting through this day, just one day at a time. Setting a short-term goal (perhaps just one meal at a time!) and meeting it is a lot more empowering than focusing on a long-term goal that you don't even know is doable yet.
- Pay attention to what your body is telling you. Appreciate the positive feedback you get from eating better and exercising that has nothing to do with the number on the scale.

- Accept that if you bring high-risk foods into your house, in all like-lihood you'll eat them. Very few people can eat just one piece of chocolate!
- Accept that if you don't have a strong plan in place for when you get hungry, there is a very good chance you'll not make the best choices. Try to eat proactively with foods you've prepared than reactively because you're overhungry.

Ultimately, what helps any one individual lose weight is to come up with her own individual portfolio of things that work. Start building your portfolio by taking stock of your past experiences. Include in your plan those things you know helped in the past (maybe shopping more consistently, exercising in the morning, not buying ice cream), and discard the things that didn't (crash dieting, diet pills, excessive exercise). Review the strategies of the NWCR successful losers and start test-driving them to see what might work for you. Ascribe to the 80/20 rule. What you do 80 percent of the time represents your habits, the things you automatically default to when your feet hit the floor in the morning. It's those habits you want to get in line. What happens 20 percent of the time or less represents what happens on days that aren't going as usual. Remember that these days don't carry anywhere near as much weight as your daily routines.

Strategy #9: Don't Go It Alone

Seek out support for your goals. A spouse, partner, family member, friend, or exercise buddy can be an invaluable asset. If you're a group person, join Weight Watchers (there are local meetings across the country, or you could try Weight Watchers online) or TOPS (Take Off Pounds Sensibly, at www.tops.org). I'm personally not a big fan of programs that require you to buy meal replacements, although that might be an option at the outset for some people. Personal coaching provided by registered dietitians can be tremendously helpful (find one in your area on the American Dietetic Association's website, at www.eatright.org). If you need a therapist to help you shake free of emotional challenges that may hold you up, by all means do it.

Because weight loss is so challenging, readiness to get involved is key. You may not be ready to actually jump into a weight-loss plan, but reading

The PCOS Diet Plan may just move you a little farther along the spectrum toward making change. Renowned University of Rhode Island psychologist James Prochaska, author of *Changing for Good*, outlines the stages that people who are able to drop bad habits tend to progress through, known as the "transtheoretical model stages of change": they are precontemplation (change isn't on your radar); contemplation (you're thinking about it and researching options); preparation (setting the stage for change); action (you're doing it!); and maintenance (you're working to make change stick).[18]

. . .

If you're not feeling ready to take charge of your health and lose weight, take some time to figure out what you need to do to establish that readiness. Each person's quest to lose weight has to be unique to their lifestyle and situation, but there are common behaviors that seem to help. The strategies outlined in this chapter are designed to help you begin to plot out your own personal plan for weight loss. If you've decided now is the time to take the pounds off, enhance your odds of success by figuring out what you need for support and find it. Support may live right under the roof with you in the form of a spouse or partner (particularly if pregnancy is your goal). Or maybe it's someone you have to seek out: a friend with similar goals, a weight-loss support group, or a registered dietitian to help you individualize your plan. It may be what you need most is a therapist with expertise in food-related issues to help you see beyond the obstacles to change. Whatever path you choose, shake off the negative self-talk that is impeding your efforts. It may not be easy to focus on the positive when trying to lose weight, but new habits and patterns are much more likely to emerge by committing to the idea that this time change is possible.

7

Taking Exercise Seriously

Whether you love it, hate it, or fall somewhere in between, you know that physical activity is an important part of a healthy lifestyle. This is particularly vital if you have polycystic ovary syndrome, because of the critical role exercise plays in managing weight, insulin resistance, and cardiovascular risk. Research demonstrates that exercise is necessary for weight loss, particularly weight-loss maintenance. Exercise increases the activity of glucose transporter 4 (GLUT 4), a protein that shuttles glucose out of the blood and into muscle and fat cells, basically acting as a natural "insulin sensitizer" for women with PCOS.[1] Exercise raises heart-healthy HDL cholesterol and lowers unhealthy LDL cholesterol and triglyceride levels commonly seen in women with PCOS. Exercise mobilizes belly fat, lowering the risk of diabetes and heart disease.[2] Regular exercise also lowers the risk of a number of cancers, Alzheimer's disease, and depression and anxiety. It improves mood and helps people remain physically independent throughout their lives.[3]

Numerous studies analyzing the benefits of exercise specific to women with PCOS have validated the importance of getting—and staying—active. Two Italian studies explored the effects of exercise on women with the syndrome (one study looked at 90 women, the other examined 124 women). Both studies divided the women into two groups, half that received a three-month structured exercise program and half who didn't. The results were that the exercisers showed significant improvement in measures of cardiovascular function and insulin resistance as well as a significant reduction in Body Mass Index (BMI) and C-reactive protein (a marker for inflammation that suggests increased risk of heart disease).[4] Another study took thirty-two women with PCOS and got them exercising for three months. They then had half the group continue to work out and the other half stop exercising for another twelve weeks. The results? Both groups showed improvement in BMI, insulin resistance, cholesterol levels, and measures of fitness after the first twelve weeks, but after twenty-four weeks the exercisers continued to improve while those who stopped exercising showed worsening of all these parameters.[5] The National Weight Control Registry participants exercise about sixty minutes a day to maintain their lost weight. Even more striking is that in people with prediabetes, eating right and exercise may lower their risk of developing diabetes by an average of 50 percent![6]

Ramping Up Your Activity

Despite what we know about the benefits of exercise, it can be hard to incorporate exercise into your life. Surveys over the past decade bear this out, showing that Americans haven't gotten any better at getting off the couch. The American College of Sport Medicine (ACSM) has long been sounding the alarm about the hazards of a sedentary lifestyle and in 2007 issued some reasonable recommendations for activity to improve health and quality of life:

- Moderately intense cardio thirty minutes a day, five days a week, or
- Vigorously intense cardio twenty minutes a day, three days a week, and
- Eight to ten strength-training exercises, eight to twelve repetitions of each exercise, twice a week.

The ACSM notes that the thirty-minute recommendation is to maintain health and lower the risk of disease, but that to lose weight and keep it off may require sixty to ninety minutes of physical activity at least five days per week.[7] In 2008 the U.S. government also got more aggressive with its exercise recommendations, issuing the first-ever "Physical Activity Guidelines for Americans," outlining exactly how much activity, and what kinds, are needed to help Americans control their weight and reduce their risk of some of the country's major health threats.[8]

In recent years thousands of studies have affirmed the benefits of physical activity for people of all ages and abilities, with very little risk. The government guidelines make recommendations for three age groups: children and adolescents, adults (including pregnant women and those with disabilities), and older adults. Daily life activity varies widely between individuals, so the recommendations focus on activities that, when added to light day-to-day activities, improve health. Examples of health-enhancing activities are brisk walking, jogging, swimming, dancing, lifting weights, and yoga. To help people rate their personal activity level, the Physical Activity Advisory Committee for the Department of Health and Human Services identified four activity categories:

- Inactive (no activity beyond baseline daily activities)
- Low (beyond baseline but less than 150 minutes a week)
- Medium (150 to 300 minutes a week)
- High (more than 300 minutes per week)

Research suggests the sweet spot for receiving consistent benefits from activity is an accumulated minimum of 150 minutes a week of moderate-intensity aerobic activities, such as walking briskly, water aerobics, ballroom and line dancing, biking on level ground or with few hills, canoeing, general gardening (raking, trimming shrubs, and so on), sports where you catch and throw (baseball, softball, volleyball), tennis (doubles). Or you can step it up and get the same benefits from seventy-five minutes of vigorous-intensity activity, such as aerobic dance, biking faster than ten miles an hour, fast dancing, heavy gardening (digging, hoeing, and so on), hiking uphill, jumping rope, martial arts (such as karate), race walking, jogging, running, doing any sport with a lot of running (basketball, hockey, soccer, and so on), swimming fast or swimming laps, and tennis (singles). Exercise more than this and it's a bonus as benefits continue to accrue as activity increases. Another helpful finding is that as little as ten minutes of activity counts toward improving your health. The guidelines also encourage muscle-strengthening activities two or more days a week to increase and preserve bone and muscle strength. Strengthening activities include weight training, resistance bands, weight-bearing calisthenics, and heavy gardening.

According to the guidelines, weight loss and preventing regain requires significantly more exercise—300 minutes or more of moderate activity per week (that's 60 minutes five days a week), or 150 "plus" minutes of vigorous activity. Most people also need to make a conscious effort to eat less when they start exercising because many people have a natural tendency to eat more, either because they're more hungry or think it's okay to reward themselves with that extra treat because they've worked out.

Accruing Your Exercise Minutes

Now that you know your numbers, how can you piece them together? Check out these ways to rack up the recommended amount of activity. For 150 minutes of moderate activity:

- Thirty minutes of brisk walking (moderate intensity) five days a week; resistance bands (strengthening) two days a week.
- Twenty-five minutes of jogging (vigorous intensity) three days a week; weight lifting two days a week.
- Thirty minutes of stationary bike or elliptical two days a week; sixty minutes of dancing one evening; thirty minutes of lawn mowing one afternoon; heavy gardening (strengthening) two days a week.
- Forty-five minutes of tennis doubles (moderate intensity) two days a week; thirty minutes of brisk walking on two days; weight machines (strength training) on two days.

For seventy-five minutes of vigorous activity:

- Sixty minutes aerobic dance on two days; fifteen minutes swimming laps one day; and lifting weights on two days.
- Thirty minutes of fast bicycling on two days; fifteen minutes of jogging one day; and weight machines on two days.

To up it to 300 minutes of moderate activity throughout the week, try these activities:

- Forty-five minutes of brisk walking daily; resistance bands on two days.
- Sixty minutes of doubles tennis on two days; sixty minutes of brisk walking on three days; and weight machines on two days.
- Forty-five minutes of stationary bike on two days; forty-five minutes of water aerobics one day; thirty minutes of bicycling on two days; sixty minutes of general gardening on one day; thirty minutes of brisk walking on two days; and resistance bands on two days.

For 150 minutes of vigorous activity a week, try these:

- Sixty minutes of aerobic dancing on two days; thirty minutes of singles tennis on one day; and weight machines on two days.
- Forty-five minutes of jogging on two days; sixty minutes of hiking one day; and weight bearing calisthenics on two days.

To determine your exercise intensity, the guidelines offer these helpful hints: When exercising moderately, you should be able to talk but not sing. During vigorous activity, you shouldn't be able to say more than a few words before breathing. You can trade off minutes by substituting one minute of vigorous activity for two minutes of moderate activity. For example, fifteen minutes of jogging (vigorous) and fifteen minutes of brisk walking (moderate) is equal to forty-five minutes of brisk walking alone.

Beyond the positive health effects of exercise, the guidelines cite additional quality-of-life reasons to increase your activity, including lower rates of depression, bringing more fun into your life, enjoyment of the outdoors, and improved body image. The guidelines also concluded that for the majority of people, the benefits of exercise far outweigh any risk—particularly if activities are varied to avoid overuse injuries—but anyone with concerns should check with her doctor first. You could also consider signing on with a personal trainer, if your budget allows. People tend to make greater gains working with a trainer because trainers tend to challenge you more than you might when exercising on your own. Trainers also provide positive feedback that may help you stick with your exercise program. Finding an exercise buddy (maybe a spouse, friend, or family member) also increases your odds of setting an exercise plan and sticking with it. For many more details on how to get your exercise routine off the ground (and couch!), check out the "Physical Activity Guidelines for Americans" website at www.health.gov/paguidelines.

. . .

What's good for managing PCOS is great for your health in general in so many ways. Both aerobic and strengthening exercises help improve your cells' use of insulin by enhancing GLUT 4 protein activity and increasing muscle density.[9] We're all familiar with the importance of exercise for weight loss and maintenance of weight loss. Not to be forgotten is the stress-relieving effect of regular exercise, which is particularly important if you're trying to manage your PCOS to undergo fertility treatments—by itself one of life's most stressful experiences. For many women, not exercising can be a source of stress because you know you should be doing it, but aren't! Becoming more active will help you feel better in your body each day, and more in control of your health.

8

Sensible Supplementation for Women with PCOS

Like most nutritionists, I take a food-first approach to meeting nutrient needs. Popping a few vitamin pills won't compensate for a poor diet, but I do think there is some sensible supplementation that most people might benefit from (whether or not they have polycystic ovary syndrome). Some nutrients can be challenging to get enough of through diet alone on a consistent basis. When I consider which supplements make sense for women with PCOS, I draw on what we know about our genetics and how humans have historically eaten. For example, human beings were genetically designed to run around naked, being exposed to the sun for much of the day; historically we had much more skin and sun exposure to synthesize "the sunshine vitamin"—vitamin D. In today's full-clothed world, most of us could use more vitamin D.

To accumulate enough carbohydrates, proteins, and fats—the nutrients we need larger amounts of to survive—the early humans hunted, gathered, picked, and dug up many different foods, each with their own unique nutrient profile, to piece together enough nutrition for survival. As a result, their diet was probably a lot more nutritionally diverse in the small nutrients—vitamins, minerals, phytonutrients, and omega-3 fats—than ours is today. The modern diet tends to be much less varied, with some people eating many of the same foods every day. Because of this, certain dietary supplements can help bring our intakes up to more desirable levels for the nutrients we should be getting more of but often aren't.

A variety of dietary supplements and herbs have been suggested, with varying degrees of scientific backing, to help manage insulin resistance and fertility. Some of these supplements show promise, while others take serious advantage of the science. My goal is to provide advice on the most studied aspects of diet and lifestyle management of PCOS, so I won't delve too much into alternative therapies. I have enough respect for herbalism to avoid dabbling in a field that is not my area of expertise, but I also believe that herbs have the potential to exert a strong medicinal effect that could possibly interact with drugs you may be taking, particularly if you're undergoing fertility treatment. Given the lack of scientific data on combining dietary supplements and herbs with fertility medications—coupled with the lack of a legal guarantee of the potency and purity of dietary supplements in the United States—I suggest avoiding anything that has not been studied sufficiently, or in doses far above the recommended levels, while trying to conceive.

The Basic Multivitamin

Most of what we call multivitamins (or "multis") are multivitamin/multimineral supplements. A good place to start is with a basic multi that provides around 100 percent of the Recommended Daily Values for a variety of vitamins and minerals. Most multis contain around 100 percent (sometimes a bit more) for the vitamins but smaller amounts of the minerals. Some minerals are bulky, so you wouldn't be able to fit a day's worth into a pill without making it prohibitively huge. Multis often only contain about 160 milligrams or so of calcium, for example, because to provide much more would bulk up the pill. For some of the minerals present in a multi, there is no established recommended dietary allowance, so no percentage of the Recommended Daily Value will appear.

If you have PCOS, there are many reasons to consider taking a daily multivitamin/multimineral supplement:

- Most women don't eat perfect diets every day, so a multi gives you a little added assurance that you've covered all the bases.
- Multis are an easy way to ensure you're getting the government-recommended minimum 400 micrograms of folic acid daily to help prevent neural tube defects in women who could become pregnant.
- Very few women get enough vitamin D, so some basic supplementation is warranted.

- Metformin, a commonly used medication to treat PCOS, may interfere with vitamin B_{12} absorption over time, so if you're on this medication, a little extra in the form of a supplement can't hurt.

Mulitvitamin/multimineral supplements also provide some magnesium, which plays a role in blood sugar regulation (crucial to the function of insulin). Multis generally only provide about 25 percent of the daily value because it is a bulky mineral. Your best bet is to include high-magnesium foods in your diet, like whole grain breads and cereals, brown rice, wheat germ, nuts, beans, spinach, artichokes, and avocados. Ideally, we'd all eat a varied enough diet not to require multis. If your diet is well balanced, by all means skip the multi and just take vitamin D and a B_{12} supplement if you're on metformin. Like most dietary supplements, multivitamin/multimineral supplements should be taken with food to enhance the absorption of the nutrients and to avoid stomach upset.

Ramping Up Your Vitamin D

Research suggests that up to 75 percent of Americans may have inadequate blood levels of vitamin D—that is, less than 30 nanograms per mil liliter (ng/ml).[1] Low levels of vitamin D are believed to be associated with higher rates of illness and death from a host of health problems, including bone disease, cardiovascular disease, diabetes, cancer, autoimmune diseases, mood disorders, and possibly other conditions.[2] Vitamin D deficiency is common because we're not designed to *eat* vitamin D as much as *synthesize* it through skin exposure to the sun. Food sources of vitamin D include fish, oysters, cheese, and egg yolks, as well as such fortified foods as milk and some juices and yogurts. The reality is, however, you'd have to eat a lot of these foods to get even the current recommendation of 400 IUs (international units) per day, which vitamin D experts have deemed too low. The Institute of Medicine is currently reviewing vitamin D requirements and is expected to issue new recommendations in the near future. Many vitamin D experts recommend 800 to 1,000 IUs of vitamin D a day for everyone not regularly exposed to the sun.[3]

Most multivitamins contain 400 IUs of vitamin D, but some are increasing their vitamin D content to 600, 800, or 1,000 IUs in anticipation of new recommendations. Calcium supplements also often contain vitamin D. Aim for a total vitamin D intake of 800 to 1,000 IUs from all supplement sources. It appears that vitamin D3 (or cholecalciferol) replenishes vitamin D levels more efficiently than vitamin D2 (ergocalciferol)— which is only about one-third as potent as vitamin D3—so look for this form on supplement labels. After two or three months have your vitamin D level checked to see if this dose is enough. The test is called a 25-hydroxyvitamin D, and a desirable blood level is 30 ng/ml or higher. Keep in mind that many people have very low vitamin D levels (below 20 ng/ml). This will need to be replaced with a big dose of vitamin D up front—often a prescription dose of 50,000 IUs of vitamin D2 (the only prescription form of vitamin D available in the United States) once a week for eight weeks—to initially ramp up the vitamin D level. After this point they may be able to settle into a maintenance dose of 1,000 IUs of vitamin D3 a day.

Research points to vitamin D as being particularly beneficial to people with insulin resistance. Accumulating research has linked low levels of vitamin D with both PCOS and metabolic syndrome, another condition where insulin resistance is a known major player, and with diabetes.[4] One study of insulin-resistant women found their insulin resistance improved after supplementing with vitamin D.[5] Given vitamin D's far-reaching positive health effects (regardless of whether it improves your PCOS), it is a supplement worth taking and a test worth having.

Considering Calcium

Women need calcium to keep our bones strong, and most women don't get enough in their diet. About 90 percent of bone mass is achieved by age eighteen in girls (age twenty in boys), but bone mass can continue to increase until around age thirty. For women, bone mass stays fairly stable from that point until menopause, after which bone loss accelerates rapidly, leaving anyone without good reserves of calcium at risk for osteoporosis. Unfortunately, fewer than 10 percent of girls between ages nine and seventeen actually get the recommended amount of calcium (1,300 milligrams a day from ages nine to eighteen).[6] Women ages nineteen to fifty need 1,000 milligrams of calcium a day, an amount that can be met with food, particularly if you like dairy products. Calcium can also be found in leafy green vegetables, broccoli, sardines, and calcium-fortified foods.

Selected Food Sources of Calcium

FOOD	MILLIGRAMS (MG) PER SERVING	PERCENT DV*
Yogurt, plain, low-fat, 8 ounces	415	42
Sardines, canned in oil, with bones, 3 ounces	324	32
Cheddar cheese, 1.5 ounces	306	31
Milk, nonfat, 8 ounces	302	30
Milk, reduced fat (2% milk fat), 8 ounces	297	30
Milk, lactose-reduced, 8 ounces**	285–302	29–30
Milk, whole (3.25% milk fat), 8 ounces	291	29
Milk, buttermilk, 8 ounces	285	29
Mozzarella, part skim, 1.5 ounces	275	28
Yogurt, fruit, low-fat, 8 ounces	245–384	25–38
Orange juice, calcium-fortified, 6 ounces	200–260	20–26
Tofu, firm, made with calcium sulfate, ½ cup***	204	20
Salmon, pink, canned, solids with bone, 3 ounces	181	18
Pudding, chocolate, instant, made with 2% milk, ½ cup	153	15
Cottage cheese, 1% milk fat, 1 cup unpacked	138	14
Tofu, soft, made with calcium sulfate, ½ cup***	138	14
Spinach, cooked, ½ cup	120	12
Ready-to-eat cereal, calcium-fortified, 1 cup	100–1,000	10–100
Instant breakfast drink, various flavors and brands, powder prepared with water, 8 ounces	105–250	10–25
Frozen yogurt, vanilla, soft serve, ½ cup	103	10
Turnip greens, boiled, ½ cup	99	10
Kale, cooked, 1 cup	94	9
Kale, raw, 1 cup	90	9
Ice cream, vanilla, ½ cup	85	8.5
Soy beverage, calcium-fortified, 8 ounces	80–500	8–50
Chinese cabbage, raw, 1 cup	74	7
Tortilla, corn, ready-to-bake/fry, 1 medium	42	4
Tortilla, flour, ready-to-bake/fry, one 6-inch diameter	37	4
Sour cream, reduced fat, cultured, 2 tablespoons	32	3
Bread, white, 1 ounce	31	3
Broccoli, raw, ½ cup	21	2
Bread, whole wheat, 1 slice	20	2
Cheese, cream, regular, 1 tablespoon	12	1

* DV = Daily Value. DVs were developed by the U.S. Food and Drug Administration to help consumers compare the nutrient contents among products within the context of a total daily diet. The DV for calcium is 1,000 mg for adults and children aged 4 and older. Foods providing 20% of more of the DV are considered to be high sources of a nutrient, but foods providing lower percentages of the DV also contribute to a healthful diet.

The U.S. Department of Agriculture's Nutrient Database website, www.nal.usda.gov/fnic/foodcomp/search, lists the nutrient content of many foods. It also provides a comprehensive list of foods containing calcium at www.nal.usda.gov/fnic/foodcomp/Data/SR20/nutrlist/sr20a301.pdf.

** Calcium content varies slightly by fat content; the more fat, the less calcium the food contains.

*** Calcium content is for tofu processed with a calcium salt. Tofu processed with other salts does not provide significant amounts of calcium.

In its food guidance system, MyPyramid, the U.S. Department of Agriculture recommends that persons aged 9 years and older eat 3 cups of foods from the milk group per day [7]. A cup is equal to 1 cup (8 ounces) of milk, 1 cup of yogurt, 1.5 ounces of natural cheese (such as Cheddar), or 2 ounces of processed cheese (such as American).

If at all possible, try to get your calcium from food sources. But if you are not a big dairy fan, or if you are lactose intolerant, you may want to take a calcium supplement. I generally recommend calcium carbonate or calcium citrate. The major difference between these two is the concentration: calcium carbonate is about 40 percent calcium and calcium citrate is about 20 percent calcium. This means you need to take more pills of citrate to get the same dose of carbonate. Like most supplements, calcium carbonate needs to be taken with food, whereas calcium citrate can be taken on an empty stomach. Calcium citrate is also more expensive. Keep in mind that for absorption, it's best to take no more than 500 milligrams of calcium at a time, so if you need more than that, take it in a divided dose at two different meals.

Preliminary research suggests there may be a connection between dairy products, dietary calcium, and weight loss, which may be one more reason to make sure you get enough through low-fat dairy foods and supplements.[7] Calorie control still trumps all when it comes to weight loss, however; there is no magic bullet. One recent study of sixty infertile women with PCOS compared the menstrual cycles of women on either calcium (1,000 milligrams) and vitamin D (400 IUs); calcium, vitamin D, and metformin; or metformin alone. The researchers found that the patients taking all three produced the most large ovarian follicles, suggesting that there might be a role for calcium and vitamin D in ovulation.[8] Again, this is only preliminary research but may provide one more reason to get enough of these two important nutrients.

Omega-3 Fats: Go Fish or Supplement

In recent years the scientific evidence supporting the importance of omega-3 fats to overall health has skyrocketed. The science for loading up on omega-3s is strongest for reducing the risk of a number of cardiovascular risk factors. Omega-3s from either fatty fish or supplements have been found to lower blood triglyceride levels and blood pressure and may slow the accumulation of cholesterol plaques in the arteries—all of which may reduce the risk of heart attack and stroke. Smaller studies suggest that omega-3s may benefit people with rheumatoid arthritis, and speculation exists about the potential benefits of omega-3s for many other diseases, including asthma, dementia, diabetes, and inflammatory bowel disease (ulcerative colitis and Crohn's disease), among others.

The three major types of omega-3 fatty acids are DHA (docosahexaenoic acid), EPA (eicosapentaenoic acid), and ALA (alpha-linolenic acid). ALA is found in seeds, green leafy vegetables, nuts, beans, and canola, flaxseed, and soybean oils. DHA and EPA are found in fatty fish (like salmon, mackerel, herring, lake trout, sardines, and tuna) and in fish oil supplements. A vegetarian source of DHA is algal oil, which fish eat to make their DHA. To get the most benefit from omega-3s, aim for fish forms. DHA and EPA are long-chain omega-3s, which are considered more physiologically active in the body. ALA is a short-chain omega-3, which needs to be converted to either DHA or EPA to be used most efficiently. Unfortunately, the human body converts very little ALA to EPA or DHA, so you're better off aiming for dietary sources of preformed DHA and EPA—fish or supplements.

DHA is critical for fetal brain and retinal development, so getting healthy amounts of this important fatty acid is important during pregnancy and breastfeeding. Getting a substantial dose of DHA may also reduce the risk of preterm delivery and possibly reduce the risk of postpartum depression.[9] Based on current intakes, most American women seem to be coming up way short on DHA, with pregnant and breastfeeding women averaging only 60 to 80 milligrams of DHA a day.[10] Experts recommend a minimum of 200 milligrams of DHA a day from either fatty fish or fish oil pills (check the label to see if a dose provides at least 200 milligrams of DHA), or algal oil pills providing this minimum dose.[11] About twelve ounces a week of fatty fish can provide enough DHA, but if you don't do this consistently, I'd err on the side of taking a daily supplement. The ceiling for safety for DHA is quite high, so don't worry about getting too much between fish and supplements.[12]

Concerns about mercury among pregnant women and those pursuing pregnancy have led to a decline in fish intake, which has contributed to abysmal DHA intakes; the worry is that mercury in fish may affect a developing baby's brain development. Ironically, this concern may potentially *contribute* to this problem by leading to low DHA levels. Women who are pregnant, or could become pregnant, should aim to eat twelve ounces of fish a week, avoiding fish high in mercury (swordfish, tilefish, king mackerel, and shark) and limiting albacore (white) tuna to no more than six ounces a week.

Other Supplements of Interest

Many women with PCOS are interested in limiting the number of pills they take as much as possible, but there are a couple of supplements to consider, particularly if you don't tolerate meds like metformin very well. Let's look at chromium picolinate and d-chiro-inositol.

Chromium Picolinate

Chromium is a trace mineral (a mineral only needed in small amounts) that plays a role in glucose regulation by sensitizing cells to the action of insulin and possibly increasing cell insulin receptor number and activity. A significant body of evidence shows that taking chromium picolinate supplements (the most common oral form) may help lower fasting blood glucose, insulin, and hemoglobin A1C levels (a measure of blood glucose control over two to three months), and increase insulin sensitivity in people with type 2 diabetes.[13] One study looking at women with PCOS and chromium found a 38 percent improvement in glucose clearance with high-dose chromium picolinate (1,000 micrograms per day).[14] But other studies don't point to the same conclusions. One recent study of patients with metabolic syndrome (caused by insulin resistance, just like PCOS) found that same 1,000-microgram dose of chromium picolinate increased the insulin response to blood glucose but did not improve other measures of glucose metabolism.[15]

People who are most likely to benefit from chromium supplementation are those who are deficient; some studies that show benefit are from China, where chromium deficiency may be more common. Unfortunately, there's no easy test to figure out whether you have a deficiency. But chromium picolinate supplements seem to be safe when taken for short periods of time. It's estimated that women need about 25 micrograms of chromium a day. The National Academy of Sciences has established a "safe and adequate daily dietary intake" range for chromium of 50 to 200 micrograms a day. If you know you have significant insulin resistance and decide to give it a try, you may want to limit it to 200 micrograms a day.[16] Most studies have used 150- to 600-microgram doses of chromium, but some studies do suggest that chromium can be safely used at doses up to 1,000 micrograms for six months. If you're trying to get pregnant, you may want to hedge your bets and limit chromium intake to around the established adequate intake (AI), about 30 micrograms a day (the amount found in multis) for women ages nineteen to thirty.

Chromium could affect your insulin metabolism, so be sure to talk to your doctor first before taking it with metformin or any other diabetes medicine. For women on thyroid medication, chromium picolinate may bind with levothyroxine (Synthroid), so you'll want to take them at least three to four hours apart.[17] Because of the lack of safety data, high-dose chromium supplements should be avoided by pregnant women or those who could become pregnant. Chromium is naturally widely distributed in the food supply in beef, chicken, seafood, eggs, whole grains, wheat germ, broccoli, apples, bananas, and spinach, but generally in small amounts. The chromium content of plant foods varies based on the chromium content of the soil it's grown in. Brewers' yeast is also a good dietary source of chromium, although it's not an easy supplement for some people to stomach.

D-Chiro-Inositol

Research shows that a deficiency of a substance involved in insulin signaling called d-chiro-inositol may contribute to the insulin resistance and hyperandrogenism seen in women with PCOS.[18] Two small studies—one using 1,200 milligrams of d-chiro-inositol once daily, the other twice a day—found that supplementing with d-chiro-inositol seemed to improve insulin sensitivity.[19] As such, some nutritionists advocate the use of d-chiro-inositol as a dietary supplement to help correct any underlying deficiency. The science in this area is definitely intriguing but still evolving, and it's not yet clear whether the research is pointing in the direction of d-chiro-inositol as a potential drug or dietary supplement.

One thing we do know is that large amounts of d-chiro-inositol are not widely available in the food supply. The most concentrated dietary source of d-chiro-inositol is buckwheat farinetta (bran), which is not easy to find in stores but, like other forms of bran, can be incorporated into oatmeal, breads, muffins, and pancakes.[20] As when introducing any new form of fiber, start slow and work your way up to allow your digestive tract to adjust. If you decide to supplement, replicating the 1,200 milligrams-plus dose of d-chiro-inositol used in studies is quite expensive. As with other supplements, because of the lack of reliable safety data, extra precaution needs to be taken with pregnancy. I'd suggest being conservative and avoiding it altogether if you are or could be pregnant.[21]

Choosing a Quality Supplement

Unlike pharmaceutical drugs, where production is overseen by the U.S. Food and Drug Administration, quality standards for production of dietary supplements in the United States is largely voluntary. Under the law dietary supplement manufacturers are supposed to be responsible for making sure their products are safe before they go to market, and that the claims on their labels are accurate and truthful. Supplements are not reviewed by the government before they're sold, however, and there have been instances where the government has stepped in and removed harmful products from the market. Here are a few things to consider when selecting a supplement:

- Is the supplement made by a large dietary supplement or pharmaceutical company? Large companies are more likely to have stringent internal production standards.
- Does it have a "USP Verified" mark on the label? The USP Dietary Supplement Verification Program is a voluntary testing and auditing program that verifies the quality, purity, and potency of dietary supplements.

• Make note of the serving size on the label, so you know how many pills you'll have to take to get the dose of nutrients listed on the label.

Above all, know what you're taking and why! I'm amazed at the number of clients I see who have no idea why they're taking a certain supplement. Also, be sure to review your supplements every year or two with a health professional. Sometimes recommendations change that might make it prudent to stop taking a particular supplement.

• • •

Dietary supplements are not going to compensate for a poorly balanced diet or lack of regular activity. It's important to keep in mind that the science of nutrition is very young, which is why recommendations seem to change on occasion. Your best bet is to eat a varied diet rich in a variety of colorful fruits and vegetables, nuts, seeds, legumes, low-fat dairy, and lean sources of animal protein. This will provide the nutrients we know are important, as well as those we *think* are important or haven't learned about yet. Beyond food, dietary supplements can be useful in making sure a few important nutrients needed for managing the cardiovascular risk and insulin resistance seen in women with PCOS—and preparing for a healthy pregnancy, if desired—are regular residents in your daily diet.

9

Reducing the Risk of Heart Disease and Diabetes

Following the recommendations of the PCOS diet plan will lower your risk of both heart disease and diabetes. The plan is designed to manage insulin resistance, which can lead to type 2 diabetes, the most common type, by replacing refined sugars and processed carbohydrates with whole grains, fruits, and vegetables, and spreading these good-quality carbs out into smaller portions over meals and snacks throughout the day. Stimulating your pancreas with smaller doses of glucose in this way lowers its workload, allowing your pancreas to preserve its insulin-secreting function. Exercise also decreases demand on the pancreas by encouraging the body's cells to use insulin more effectively, so your pancreas won't feel compelled to keep churning it out.

The combined approach of controlling portions of carbs, watching fat intake, filling up on lean proteins, eating more fruits, vegetables, and whole grains, and increasing activity is consistent with what we know helps people lose weight and keep it off. This is the single most potent thing anyone can do to reduce his or her risk of diabetes. As individuals, and as a society as a whole, we need to do *everything possible* to reduce the incidence and health risks of diabetes, the costs of which are imposing an unsustainable burden on the country's health-care system.

The Menace of Metabolic Syndrome

Because diabetes and cardiovascular disease are so tightly linked, reducing the risk of one disease generally helps cut the risk of the other. Unfortunately, a large chunk of the U.S. population is well on the road to developing both of these conditions. Whereas PCOS affects only women, it's estimated that more than fifty million American men and women (approaching one-fifth of the population) have metabolic syndrome, another condition driven by insulin resistance that's characterized by the following collection of cardiovascular risk factors:

- Abdominal obesity (excessive "belly fat")
- Abnormal blood fat and cholesterol levels—high triglycerides, low HDL cholesterol, and high LDL cholesterol—that encourage plaque buildup in artery walls
- High blood pressure
- Insulin resistance
- Prothrombotic state, or a tendency for the blood to clot more easily
- Proinflammatory state, often diagnosed with a C-reactive protein test, a marker for inflammation in the blood

All of these risk factors can be positively affected by the PCOS diet plan. The primary goal of the plan is to reduce insulin resistance and circulating levels of insulin—big contributors to metabolic syndrome and heart disease. Controlling insulin resistance with diet and exercise helps reduce belly fat. Avoiding saturated and trans fats and limiting intake of sweets helps to improve triglyceride and cholesterol levels and enhance insulin sensitivity. Losing weight, exercising regularly, and adding fruits, vegetables, whole grains (plus small amounts of nuts to the diet) can help lower blood pressure. Increasing your intake of omega-3 fats can help thin the blood and reduce inflammation inside the cardiovascular system.

The American Heart Association defines metabolic syndrome as the presence of three or more of these criteria:

- Elevated waist circumference:
    Men—equal to or greater than 40 inches (102 centimeters)
    Women—equal to or greater than 35 inches (88 centimeters)
- Elevated triglycerides: equal to or greater than 150 milligrams per deciliter (mg/dl)
- Reduced HDL cholesterol (the "good" kind):
    Men—less than 40 mg/dl
    Women—less than 50 mg/dl

- Elevated blood pressure: equal to or greater than 130/85 mm Hg
- Elevated fasting glucose: equal to or greater than 100 mg/dl[1]

Whether you have PCOS, metabolic syndrome, or suffer from even one of these criteria, controlling these numbers is an important part of protecting your cardiovascular system. What should *your* goal numbers be? As a means of monitoring cardiovascular risk, a primary care physician will monitor your blood pressure, cholesterol profile, and fasting blood glucose to see if your numbers are drifting into a higher-risk range. Below I've outlined the range of where your goal numbers should fall for total cholesterol, HDL, LDL, triglycerides, blood pressure, and fasting blood glucose; you'll see what are considered moderate and high elevations. Keep in mind that although a diagnosis of metabolic syndrome requires you to have at least three risk factors for heart disease, having even one number out of range should trigger you to reexamine and revamp your diet and lifestyle habits.

Total cholesterol:
- Under 200 mg/dl is desirable
- 200–239 mg/dl is borderline high risk
- 240 mg/dl or higher is high risk

HDL ("good" cholesterol):
- A level of 60 or higher offers some protection against heart disease

LDL ("bad" cholesterol):
- Optimal: less than 100 mg/dl
- Near/above optimal: 100–129 mg/dl
- Borderline high: 130–159 mg/dl
- High: 160–189 mg/dl
- Very high: 190 mg/dl or above

Triglycerides (fat in your blood):
- Normal: less than 150 mg/dl
- Borderline high: 150–199 mg/dl
- High: 200–499 mg/dl
- Very high: 500 mg/dl[2]

Blood pressure:
- Normal: less than 120 systolic, less than 80 diastolic
- Prehypertension: 120–139 systolic, 80–89 diastolic
- Hypertension: 140 or higher systolic, 90 or higher diastolic[3]

Fasting blood glucose (after at least an eight-hour fast):
- Normal: below 100 mg/dl
- Prediabetes: 100–125 mg/dl
- Diabetes: 126 mg/dl or above[4]

DASH toward a Healthier Heart

According to Tufts University nutrition researcher Margo Woods, the most comprehensive and effective dietary approach to lowering your cardiovascular risk is to follow the DASH diet. DASH stands for Dietary Approaches to Stop Hypertension but actually encompasses all the recommendations for a heart-healthy diet.[5]

The DASH diet is a comprehensive eating plan based on research funded by the National Heart Lung and Blood Institute that found that adding foods to the diet that are rich in nutrients known to affect blood pressure (and other heart-health factors) can reduce it in as little as two weeks. DASH is low in total fat, saturated fat, and cholesterol, and emphasizes fruits, vegetables, and fat-free or low-fat milk and milk products. It includes whole grains, fish, poultry, and small portions of nuts, seeds, and legumes. This diet combination is rich in potassium, magnesium, calcium, lean protein, and fiber—all dietary elements known to keep blood pressure down. DASH also recommends limiting sodium to about 2,300 milligrams per day (the equivalent of one teaspoon), as sodium can affect blood pressure. DASH is a high-carb plan—about 55 percent of daily calories—which is a little higher than in the PCOS diet plan, but with attention to carb portions the two plans can easily interface. This might be in order if you have high blood pressure and/or high cholesterol in addition to PCOS. Based on a sample 1,600-calorie diet (which would encourage weight loss in most women), DASH recommends a daily intake as outlined in the chart that follows.

The DASH Diet (1,600 calories)

FOOD GROUP	SERVINGS PER DAY
Grains	6 servings
Vegetables	3 to 4 servings
Fruits	4 servings
Fat-free or 1 percent milk or milk products	2 to 3 servings
Lean meats, poultry, and fish	3 to 6 ounces
Nuts, seeds, and legumes	3 servings a week
Fats and oils	2 servings
Sweets and added sugars	0 (higher-calorie levels allow no more than 5 servings per week)

Compared to these DASH recommendations, you may be eating a little more lean protein (six to eight ounces a day) and a little less carbohydrate, but that's okay. I'd suggest trimming the grain portions first and really emphasizing whole grains to get the benefit of the minerals. As a woman with PCOS, you have the added concern of managing insulin resistance, which isn't good for your heart, so merging the best of both plans is probably the strongest approach. And don't forget exercise! It's one of the strongest lifestyle strategies there is for controlling both blood pressure and insulin resistance.

• • •

Polycystic ovary syndrome presents a lifelong threat to cardiovascular health and risk of diabetes. Research suggests that women with the condition have four to seven times the risk of heart attack than women of the same age without PCOS. They have a greater risk of developing high blood pressure as well, and upwards of 50 percent will have diabetes or prediabetes by age forty.[6] Fortunately, following the PCOS diet plan will trickle down to benefit these other health concerns as it helps to manage insulin resistance and weight. It's no coincidence that the PCOS diet plan also includes many of the elements of the heart-healthy DASH diet.[7]

PART 3

The PCOS Diet: Making It Happen

10

Eating the PCOS Diet Way: Meals and Snacks

Now that you understand *why* and *how* the PCOS diet plan will help you manage your PCOS and improve your health, it's time to decide *which* carbohydrate-distributed diet option is best for you: the balanced-plate approach (because it starts with general changes and doesn't feel too threatening) or the carb-counting option (because you feel you need more structure). But how do you actually put these plans into daily practice?

The first step is to budget some time into your week to focus on food—planning what you're going to buy, shopping, preparing meals, and packing them to travel with you if necessary. For most people this requires shuffling around some priorities, but it won't always feel so hard. As your diet and lifestyle evolves to a new place, tasks that feel like work at the outset will eventually become your "new normal." Your grocery cart will look different, and you may add a few key culinary pieces of equipment to your kitchen. (If you don't already have an electric countertop grill, get one!) But like learning anything new, you need to do your homework and practice, practice, practice. The meal and snack ideas offered throughout this chapter are designed to ease your way toward healthier eating. As you get good at reading food labels and integrating a few new recipes or food combinations into your usual repertoire, things will settle into a fresh routine of PCOS-friendly habits that will improve your health and help you feel better about your body.

Making Meals a Priority

If the desired outcome is that most days you eat pretty well, you have to figure out what you need to do to set the stage for that to happen. Let's look at the process of eating well as a domino effect, where the last domino to fall is "I ate a good meal." We'll track it backward to see what steps need to occur to make that final step happen:

- If you want to eat well, you have to have some good food choices close at hand.
- To have those healthy foods as your default choices, you need to make time to prepare your meals and snacks. Pack them up if they are going to work with you.
- To have healthy foods to prepare and pack, you need to budget some time each week for shopping at the grocery store or farmers' market, so that good food options are readily available for you. Share this responsibility with a spouse, partner, family member, or friend.
- To have time available to shop, you need to decide how to plan the rest of your time to prioritize food shopping throughout the week.

This planning part eludes many would-be weight losers. To make it happen, you have to decide this step is important. You have to *know* that making healthy changes and adjustments in your diet and lifestyle is possibly the most important thing you need to accomplish in your life right now—particularly if part of your plan is getting pregnant and time is of the essence.

For many of us, if we don't take time to think about our next meal, and try to plan dinner when we're starving, the chances of grabbing takeout or making boxed macaroni and cheese are pretty high. That doesn't mean you have to start cooking elaborate, gourmet meals every night from scratch, though. I'm all for shortcuts as long as they result in reasonable choices. Unless you married a chef, or are wealthy enough to hire one, you need to put at least a little elbow grease into planning and preparing meals. Our ancestors devoted much of their time to figuring out what they were going to eat and how they were going to get it on the table. Since the beginning of recorded history, food procurement and preparation was a valued life skill passed down from one generation to the next.

Think about it: If you have some basic cooking skills, someone probably taught you them when you were young. This point is particularly important if there are children in your household: if no one under your roof is cooking, how is the next generation supposed to figure out how to feed themselves when they're out on their own? They won't. They'll eat out *all* the time, which is more expensive and likely to feed the ever-inflating obesity epidemic in this country. So, if nothing else, consider your efforts to prepare meals at home—at least *most* of the time—as an investment in the next generation! Let's walk through the day—meal by meal—and review some simple suggestions to help make meal planning go a little smoother.

Begin with Breakfast

It's not called the most important meal of the day for nothing. If you want to control your insulin resistance and lose weight, you simply have to eat breakfast. If the food choice is a healthy one and stays within your carb budget, there's a lot of room for flexibility. Make sure you budget ten to fifteen minutes into your morning, either at home or at work, to make breakfast happen. If you're trying to eat mindfully, you would not be eating while driving (this is potentially dangerous too!), running around your house, or during a stressful meeting. Regardless, what matters most is that you eat a breakfast, and one that you eat at home or bring to work is going to be a better choice than the pastries or giant-size muffins you'd get at a local coffee shop or be offered at a breakfast meeting.

There are four typical mistakes people make at breakfast time. Do you make any of these?

1. Skipping breakfast! After more than twenty years of counseling thousands of people on weight loss, I'm here to tell you that skipping breakfast is the kiss of death to weight-loss efforts. Studies show that people who skip breakfast tend to eat more at night, which is a common contributor to weight gain.

2. Thinking that coffee with cream and sugar or artificial sweetener is breakfast. It's not! I have no problem with including coffee with low-fat milk and a little bit of sweetener with your breakfast, but it doesn't add the valuable nutrients you need to kick off your day.

3. Grabbing breakfast where you get your coffee. There are rarely healthy choices available in a grab-and-go coffee shop. A donut is the obvious poor choice, but don't assume the other options are much better: the bagels, muffins, and scones often in the display case are usually way too big—typically double or even triple a single serving size.

4. Making the excuse that you don't have time. If you have time to pull into a coffeehouse parking lot, stand in line, wait for your beverage, prep it, and walk back to your car, you can find ten minutes to grab a quick breakfast at home before you leave the house.

Healthy Breakfast Options

Assume you're working with a 45- to 60-gram carb budget and want to work in a protein source. Even though the diabetes exchange lists count 8 ounces of milk as 12 grams of carb, we're using 15 grams for simplicity's sake. You also may opt for a slightly smaller 30-gram carb breakfast, but you want to make sure you get enough carbs to keep your blood glucose levels in a stable range until your midmorning snack or lunch.

Healthy Breakfast Options

BREAKFAST CHOICE	CARBS (GRAMS)	
One whole wheat English muffin	30	
1 tablespoon peanut or other nut butter	0	**45 grams total**
8 ounces 1 percent or skim milk	15	
Two slices whole wheat toast (15 grams each)	30	
Half cup 1 percent or nonfat cottage cheese	0	**60 grams total**
8 ounces 1 percent or skim milk	15	
One-third cantaloupe	15	
One whole wheat English muffin	30	
One egg or one serving egg substitute (combined with English muffin as an egg sandwich)	0	**45 grams total**
1 tablespoon tub spread	0	
8 ounces 1 percent or skim milk	15	

Healthy Breakfast Options, continued

BREAKFAST CHOICE	CARBS (GRAMS)	
One whole wheat waffle	15	
1 tablespoon peanut or other nut butter	0	**45 grams total**
One small banana	15	
8 ounces 1 percent or skim milk	15	
One (six-inch) whole wheat tortilla	15	
One egg scrambled and cooked with nonstick spray and a slice of reduced-fat cheese	0	**45 grams total**
One pear	15	
8 ounces 1 percent or skim milk	15	
1 cup cooked old-fashioned or steel-cut oatmeal	30	
1 tablespoon chopped walnuts	0	**45 grams total**
2 tablespoons dried cranberries or raisins	15	
6 ounces plain or artificially sweetened yogurt	15	
1/4 cup low-fat granola	15	
1 tablespoon chopped nuts	0	**45 grams total**
Half cup canned pineapple (in water)	15	
3/4 cup dry whole grain cereal	15	
2 tablespoons dried fruit	15	
1–2 tablespoons chopped nuts (mix all together)	0	**45 grams total**
One hard-boiled egg	0	
8 ounces 1 percent or skim milk	15	

Mind-Set Intervention: Assume That Change Is Possible!

I get that people are busy in the morning. I am too. It's not always easy. I may be eating cereal with one hand and putting on makeup with the other, but I make sure breakfast always happens. You just have to give yourself a chance to establish the habit. If you typically skip breakfast, start with a small change: grab a piece of fruit or a granola bar to snap your metabolism out of hibernation mode. A next step might be budgeting in some extra time: set your alarm just ten minutes earlier! Then you can work on the specific food choice.

But what if you don't like traditional breakfast foods? Try these tasty alternatives instead—just be sure to eat something!

BREAKFAST CHOICE	CARBS (GRAMS)	
Two slices whole grain bread	30	
Two slices reduced-fat cheese (melted on top)	0	**45 grams total**
One apple	15	
One (six-inch) whole wheat tortilla	15	
2 ounces leftover chicken	0	
17 grapes (roughly a fistful)	15	**40–42 grams total**
6 ounces sugar-free hot chocolate	10–12 grams (check the food label)	
Ten Ak-Mak stone ground sesame crackers	38 (2 servings per the food label)	
Two Laughing Cow spreadable cheese wedges	0	**53 grams total**
4 ounces orange juice	15	
1 ounce (30 grams) whole grain crackers	15–20 (the number of crackers varies by type—check the food label)	
1/3 cup hummus	15	**45 grams total**
One small orange	15	
One small bagel (such as Original Lender's frozen)	30	
One slice turkey	0	
One slice cheese	0	**45 grams total**
1 teaspoon light mayonnaise or mustard	0	
Lettuce and tomato	0	
8 ounces 1 percent or skim milk	15	

Any of these breakfast suggestions could be trimmed by fifteen grams of carb by transporting some of the breakfast carbs to a midmorning snack. Here's another option for those who prefer a smaller breakfast while they're waiting for their digestive tract to wake up: enjoy half of your breakfast first thing in the morning and the other half as a midmorning snack. Or it could be two-thirds at breakfast and one-third at midmorning snack time. Experiment with the timing: there is enough flexibility in the plan to make it work for you.

Midmorning: To Snack or Not to Snack?

The answer to this question depends on two things: (1) how filling was your breakfast, and (2) how hungry will you be by lunch if you don't snack? You want to approach your next meal or snack when you're maybe hungry but not starving. On a hunger scale of one to ten, you want to hit the next meal or snack when you're at a five or six, not an eight or ten. One way to up the odds of making it to lunch without always needing a snack is to ramp up the breakfast protein. Adding eggs, low-fat cottage cheese, or Greek yogurt (which is higher in protein than regular yogurt) to your breakfast may leave you feeling more satisfied and less in need of a snack. Studies have also shown oatmeal (not the sugary kind) to be super-satisfying, keeping hunger at bay for a longer period of time.

But if you *do* need a midmorning snack, by all means have one. Because breakfast and lunch are generally much closer together than lunch and dinner, though, try limiting this snack to a piece of fruit if possible. Most people don't eat enough fruit, so checking one off midmorning fulfills half your requirement (at least two a day) by lunch. In my experience some insulin-resistant women need a protein-carb snack midmorning to head into lunch without getting overly hungry. Maybe an apple and four to five almonds will do it in the morning, whereas something more substantial may be needed in the afternoon.

Let's Do Lunch!

First and foremost, don't skip lunch! This can be a full-blown setup for reactive overeating that begins in front of the vending machine at 4 p.m. and doesn't stop until you fall into bed. I'm a stickler for eating pattern. Even if lunch has to start as a half-lunch grabbed at your desk before a meeting, do it. It's better than waiting until later when you're overhungry (at an eight to ten) and no longer in very good control of what you eat. You might think about flipping lunch and dinner, so lunch is the larger meal. This may help you control your hunger for the rest of the day, and load you down with fewer calories at night. My grandparents, who both lived to a ripe old age, called lunch "dinner," implying it was the main meal of the day (and people were a lot thinner back then!).

Some people do better with this eating pattern: breakfast in the morning, half of their lunch at noon, the other half at 3 or 4 p.m., and dinner by around 7 p.m. They're basically having a meal or mini-meal every four hours or so. Same number of calories, evenly distributed throughout the day, with decent portions of protein with each eating episode. Why not try this pattern and see how you feel?

Don't make the plant part of your lunch an afterthought. Find a way to work both fruits and vegetables into at least half of your meal. You'll walk away feeling a lot fuller on fewer calories. If you're bringing lunch from home, make it the night before while you're cleaning the kitchen and not settled in yet for the night. Waiting until morning increases the odds that you'll become busy and scrap the idea. If you can't pack a lunch to take to work, make the most of your options, whether it be the employee cafeteria or a local sandwich shop. Look for places that allow you to piece together a decent lunch a la carte. A healthy salad bar can't be beat. Follow these guidelines: select five vegetables (reflecting a variety of colors), two to three added proteins (grilled chicken, half a hard-boiled egg, and a small sprinkling of grated or crumbled cheese works nicely), and a tablespoon of raisins or dried cranberries for texture and a touch of sweetness. Top your salad with half a ladle of low-cal dressing for a calorie-controlled, satisfying lunch. The choices may not be perfect, but the decision making may be less challenging than the corner deli.

These are the five most common mistakes people make at lunchtime. Do you see yourself in any of these?

1. Skipping lunch altogether.
2. Getting busy with work and eating lunch too late (when you're at an eight to ten on the hunger scale), at which point you're at high risk for reactive overeating.
3. Eating too little to hold you over for a decent amount of time. A salad with too little protein, fat-free dressing, and pita bread will not fill the void in your stomach for long.
4. Going into business lunches starving, when you're at high risk for grabbing a huge sandwich, bag of chips, and a Frisbee-sized cookie—a carb overload disaster for women with PCOS.
5. Being unrealistic about the challenges of eating healthfully in a restaurant. Sandwiches are typically twice the size they should be, and there's often a lot more hidden fat in meals than you realize or

can easily identify. This doesn't mean you can't enjoy the occasional dining out for lunch, but be a realist.

What's on the Lunch Menu?

As at breakfast time, aim for a forty-five- to sixty-gram carbohydrate budget for lunch. Remember: Nonstarchy vegetables are so low in carbohydrate, they are considered a write-off, so the carb count will be zero. Because lunch and dinner are fairly far apart for most people, including a three- to four-ounce portion of protein with lunch will slow the movement of food out of the stomach and complicate digestion, helping to steady your blood glucose levels and keep you feeling fuller longer. Three ounces of cooked protein is about the size of a deck of cards. Four ounces is about the size of a hockey puck.

Plan for the plant part of the meal. Vegetables can be raw in the form of a salad, whole carrots, sliced peppers, or a celery stalk (or any other vegetable you like raw); or they can be cooked—as a broth-based vegetable soup or leftover reheated vegetables from the night before. Your fruit servings can be in the form of a raw piece of fruit, a serving of fruit salad, or a couple of tablespoons of dried fruit sprinkled into a salad. Watch those added fats, though—something that's more challenging if you're eating out a lot. The usual offenders are mayonnaise (100 calories per tablespoon), too much full-fat salad dressing (these can be 80 to 180 calories per two-tablespoon serving), too much cheese, sandwiches grilled in too much butter, cream soups, and french fries.

Throughout the list of lunch options below I'll point out "free" and "combination foods" from the diabetic exchange lists. You can see why some foods that have small amounts of carb are counted as free, and other less obvious choices count either all or in part as a carb (like broth-based soup, for example). Nonstarchy vegetables are considered freebies, so we count their carbs as "zero." We're working with estimates here, so don't sweat the small stuff!

Healthy Lunch Options

LUNCH CHOICE	CARBS (GRAMS)	
Two slices whole wheat bread (15 grams per slice)	30	**60 grams total**
Two slices turkey, one slice cheese	0	
2 teaspoons low-fat mayonnaise	0	
Lettuce and tomato	0	
8 ounces 1 percent or skim milk	15	
17 grapes (a handful)	15	
Half (six-inch) whole wheat pita	15	**45 grams total** (*Up to this amount is free on the exchange list.)
2 ounces lean roast beef, one slice cheese	0	
2 teaspoons barbecue sauce*	0	
Romaine lettuce, sliced red peppers	0	
One pear	15	
8 ounces skim or 1 percent milk	15	
One slice whole wheat bread	15	**45 grams total** ^ = 1 carb "combination food" ** = negligible carb, 1.5 tablespoons = 1 carb; 1 tablespoon of low-fat dressing is free, the other tablespoon contributes marginal amount of carb.)
1 tablespoon peanut butter	0	
1 teaspoon 100 percent fruit spread*	0	
1 cup chicken noodle soup*	15	
1 cup baby carrots and chopped celery	0	
2 tablespoons low-fat dressing for dipping**	0	
One apple	15	
Lettuce, tomato, cukes, onions, peppers, and so on	0	**45 grams total**
3 ounces grilled chicken	0	
Half cup kidney or garbanzo beans	15	
2 tablespoons low-fat dressing	0	
Half (six-inch) whole wheat pita	15	
One packet sugar-free instant hot chocolate	15	
One small hamburger or cheeseburger	0	**45 grams total** (*Up to this amount is free on the exchange list.)
One small bun	30	
1 tablespoon ketchup*	0	
Side salad with low-fat dressing	0	
8 ounces skim or 1 percent milk	15	

Healthy Lunch Options, continued

LUNCH CHOICE	CARBS (GRAMS)	
Two slices whole grain bread	30	**45 grams total**
Two slices cheese (melted on top in toaster oven)	0	
One slice tomato (on top of cheese; sprinkle with Italian herbs)	0	
1 cup baby carrots	0	
Half cup fruit cocktail in juice or water	15	
Sugar-free beverage	0	
Quarter (twelve-inch) cheese pizza	30	**60 grams total** *(Note: The kidney beans add protein and fiber to the salad for satiety.)*
Side salad with low-cal dressing	0	
Half cup kidney beans (pour on the salad)	15	
One orange	15	
Sugar-free beverage	0	
2 cups bean soup (lentil, pea, black bean)	30	**60 grams total** *(Note: The bean soup also counts as protein.)*
One small roll	15	
Two small plums	15	
Water or sugar-free beverage	0	
One small (six-inch) sub roll	30–45	**45–60 grams total**
3 ounces turkey, ham, or roast beef	0	
Lettuce, tomato, onions, peppers, pickles	0	
1–2 teaspoons mustard or low-fat mayo	0	
8 ounces skim or 1 percent milk	15	
³/₄ cup 1 percent cottage cheese (equals 3 ounces of protein)	0	**45 grams total**
1 ounce (30 grams) of whole grain crackers	15	
1 cup cubed cantaloupe	15	
Two small (2¹/₄-inch-wide) chocolate chip cookies	15	
Water or sugar-free beverage	0	
One (six-inch) whole wheat tortilla	15	**60 grams total**
¹/₄ cup tabouli	(negligible carbs)	
Half cup black beans	15	
Roasted red pepper slices	0	
¹/₃ cup shredded part-skim cheese	0	
One apple	15	
8 ounces skim or 1 percent milk	15	

Healthy Lunch Options, continued

LUNCH CHOICE	CARBS (GRAMS)	
2 tablespoons peanut butter	0	**45 grams total** *(Note: The added sugar per serving in the peanut butter is negligible.)*
1 ounce (30 grams) whole grain crackers	15	
1 cup tomato soup	15	
Carrot and celery sticks	0	
8 ounces skim or 1 percent milk	15	
One medium baked potato	30	**60 grams total**
1 cup chili	30	
1/4 cup shredded part-skim cheese	0	
Side salad with low-cal dressing	0	
Water or sugar-free beverage	0	
3–4 ounces chicken or shrimp	0	**60 grams total**
1 cup stir-fried vegetables	0	
1/3 cup brown rice or white rice	15	
One egg roll (half if eaten with duck sauce)	30	
Half cup pineapple chunks	15	

Salad Specifics

If you stick with vegetable-only ingredients at the salad bar, salads are an excellent filler, helping you feel like you've eaten a lot while actually consuming very few calories. Focusing on vegetables only is critical because fat-laden add-ons with little nutritional value have the potential to crank up the calories. Things to avoid (or use very little of) in your salads are croutons, bacon bits, pasta salad, potato salad, large amounts of cheese, and oil-based bean salads. Healthy-fat choices worthy of a small sprinkle on your salad (roughly a teaspoon or two at the most) are nuts, seeds, olives, and soy nuts.

Follow this golden rule when assembling a salad: it must contain at least five ingredients. That's at least four vegetables and a sprinkling of some sort of protein (beans, nuts, or reduced-fat cheese). You may add to that a teaspoon or two of dried cranberries or raisins for added nutrients, interest, and texture. Many of the health-promoting nutrients in vegetables are the pigments that give them their color, so when you look at your salad you want to see a variety of color: deep green lettuce, red tomatoes, yellow peppers, black olives, orange carrots, and light green cucumbers. Visual appeal matters!

Avoid drowning your salad in dressing. The universal portion is two tablespoons, but be sure to measure it out (it's easy to go overboard when pouring from the bottle). Compare the calories—some full-fat varieties contain more than two hundred calories in two tablespoons, whereas low-fat varieties can be far less. I'm a fan of using smaller amounts of low-fat salad dressing versus larger amounts of fat-free for two reasons: (1) they tend to taste better and (2) the fat in the dressing helps us digest many of the fat-soluble phytonutrients found in plant foods. Preferably, the fat source in the dressing would be heart-healthy olive or canola oil, which can count for your small amount of healthful fat included in the meal. Not a big fan of bottled dressings? By all means, make your own! You could also try using dry salad dressing packets that come with a glass bottle, where you choose your source of vinegar (I prefer balsamic) and oil (use a little of both olive and canola and the fat won't solidify in the fridge), and follow the directions for "less oil" dressing.

Healthy Midafternoon Snacks

Not everyone needs an afternoon snack, but most people who struggle with portion control need something to fill the void during that long stretch between lunch and dinner. This is particularly important given that for many of us dinnertime is a lot later than it used to be. If lunch is at noon or 1 p.m. and dinner is at 7 or 8 p.m., hunger can really start to mount by around 3 or 4 p.m.

It can't be stated enough that weight control is about calories, so the goal of incorporating an afternoon snack is to help keep hunger under control so dinner is not twice the size of every other meal of the day. Even if your afternoon snack is 250 calories, they're calories well spent if it prevents you from overeating 600 calories at dinner. The key is to plan for a balanced snack that includes a portion of carbohydrate (to keep your blood glucose levels from dipping and triggering carb cravings) and a portion of lean protein (to help steady glucose levels and help you feel full).

Eating Nuts without Going Nuts

Despite years of being on the "bad food" list because of their fat content, most people are now aware that in small amounts nuts can be an important part of a healthy diet. They're a good source of fiber, plant protein, healthful monounsaturated fat, vitamins, and minerals. They also happen to be 80 percent fat, so portion control is key if you're trying to lose weight. Rather than mindlessly noshing on nuts in front of the TV, a better approach is to incorporate small amounts of nuts into foods: sprinkle them on cereals or salads, mix them into a homemade trail mix, or stir them into yogurt. To avoid calorie overload—which is incredibly easy to do with nuts—I generally recommend limiting nuts to half-ounce portions and pairing them with a carb for a snack. Check out this list to see what a half ounce of your favorite nuts looks like:

Nut Portion Sizes and Calories

NUT	NUTS PER ½ OUNCE	CALORIES PER ½ OUNCE
Almonds	11	85
Brazil nuts	3–4	93
Cashews	9	81
Hazelnuts	10	89
Macadamia nuts	5–6	102
Peanuts	14	83
Pecans	10	100
Pine nuts	1½ tablespoons	72
Pistachio nuts	23	81
Walnuts	7 halves	93

Peanut butter and other nut butters are also healthy additions to the diet as long as you're mindful of portions: nut butters average around a hundred calories per tablespoon. Think about how easy it is to lick that off a knife. If there was ever a food to measure, this is it!

Healthy Snack Suggestions

Being prepared is an important part of establishing healthy eating habits. Load up on snack baggies (half-size storage bags); small plastic containers for things like hummus, peanut butter, and low-fat salad dressings; and an

A Word about Crackers

When you look at the nutrition label of a box of crackers, you'll notice that the serving sizes vary considerably depending on whether the crackers are tiny (like oyster crackers) or big (like graham crackers). With few exceptions crackers are portioned out in one-ounce servings, which the labels usually list as roughly thirty grams (by weight). Because crackers alone aren't very filling, and starting to eat them alone can easily escalate into eating too many, I recommend pairing a half a serving (half an ounce) of crackers with a protein, like reduced-fat cheese or cottage cheese, tuna mixed with light mayo, or a small amount of peanut butter. In general, a half-ounce serving of crackers is about ten grams of carb, which is close enough to our fifteen-gram carb portions that I'd just consider it a carb choice. Be sure to choose crackers with at least two grams of fiber, suggesting there are some whole grains in there, roughly three grams of fat (so you know they're low fat), and no trans fats.

insulated lunch bag and ice pack to carry it all to work. Experiment with these afternoon snack ideas, or use them as a blueprint for a snack you'll find satisfying:

- Half cup 1 percent cottage cheese and half cup canned fruit (in water or juice)
- Half cup cottage cheese flavored with herb seasoning and a half ounce of crackers
- Half cup tuna mixed with light mayo and a half ounce of crackers
- 1¹/₂ tablespoons peanut butter and a half ounce of crackers
- 1¹/₂ tablespoons peanut butter on a sliced apple or small banana
- Two wedges of Laughing Cow Light spreadable cheese and a half ounce of crackers
- Two wedges Laughing Cow Light spreadable cheese on four crackers, carrots and celery sticks
- 1 ounce reduced-fat hard cheese (like Cabot 50 percent reduced fat) with a half ounce of crackers
- One small whole wheat pita filled with 2 tablespoons hummus
- Half a ham-and-cheese sandwich with mustard on whole wheat bread or a small whole wheat pita
- Half an English muffin topped with 1 tablespoon pizza sauce and grated part-skim mozzarella, heated in the toaster oven

- One slice whole grain bread with one slice reduced-fat cheese, heated in the toaster oven
- 6 ounces light yogurt and a half ounce of nuts
- One light or plain yogurt mixed with 2 tablespoons low-fat granola
- Half ounce of nuts and one fruit
- One to two slices of turkey rolled into a small tortilla or stuffed into a pita with lettuce, tomato, and/or sliced red peppers
- One hard-boiled egg and a half ounce of crackers or one slice wheat toast
- 6 ounces nonfat or low-fat Greek yogurt (almost three times the protein content of regular yogurt and less added sugar)
- Half cup high-fiber cereal with 4 ounces skim or 1 percent milk
- One reduced-fat cheddar stick or string cheese with half-ounce serving of crackers or a fruit
- $3/4$ cup homemade trail mix, made with 2 cups high-fiber cereal, $1/3$ cup chopped nuts, and $1/3$ cup dried fruit (makes about $3^1/2$ servings)
- One hard granola bar coated with 2 teaspoons peanut butter

Notice that I haven't included things like cereal bars and chewy granola bars in this list. They tend to be low in fiber and protein and often high in sugar. Also, be wary of hundred-calorie packs of crackers, chips, or cookies. They're only worth a hundred calories if you eat just one pack! The cracker packs could be paired with a protein, but don't expect a hundred-calorie pack of cookies to do much to hold you over. They're also expensive. Mini-packs may be a better option for that occasional aftermeal treat, particularly because they lack any valuable nutrients. Make sure you factor in the carbs if you have these treats at the end of a meal.

What's for Dinner?

The number-one rule about dinner is don't eat it too late! This tends to encourage reactive overeating at the worst time of day to overload on calories. Eating too much at night can kill your appetite for breakfast, reinforcing a bad habit of skipping this important meal. Preparing balanced-plate dinners most nights of the week is one of your most important behavioral tasks. Even if you're not yet convinced you need to do this for yourself, if children are in your life (or your future), you absolutely need to model healthy eating for their sake. Children learn what they live, and eating out all the time or not eating until you're starving is an outright recipe for overeating and becoming overweight.

Don't feel like you need to be a gourmet cook to make a decent dinner. I'm a huge fan of cooking in bulk. If you're going to make chicken or pork chops, make enough for three meals. Make enough brown rice at the beginning of the week to have extra to reheat in the microwave (for more flavorful brown rice, try cooking it in low-fat chicken broth instead of water). Stock your refrigerator with frozen vegetables so you always have something if you run out of the preferred fresh veggies. Make chili, soups, stews, and other meals you can prepare in a big batch and freeze in single-serving portions. All you have to do is thaw, heat, and serve with a salad. It doesn't have to be fancy! If cookbooks intimidate you, buy one of those photo albums with the tear-back plastic pages and collect your own recipes from cooking and lifestyle magazines or online recipe websites. Whenever you eat something you like at someone's house or party, ask the host for the recipe and put it in your book. The only rule I suggest is to prepare it first so you know you like it. Accumulating your own collection of recipes you enjoy gives you something to flip through the next time you need inspiration.

When preparing dinner, think vegetables first, not last. Although it's natural to start planning with the protein part of the meal, don't let vegetables be an afterthought. Using the balanced-plate approach, half your plate should be vegetables. Having them in your house in fresh, frozen, or canned (in a pinch) form is key to making them a priority. If getting to the store is a challenge, consider a trial of home-delivered groceries. I've found this to be a great option for busy people. Not confident in your culinary skills? Consider taking a cooking class through a local adult education center. Culinary schools sometimes offer classes for the community.

Here are the three most common mistakes people make at dinnertime. Do you see yourself in any of these?

1. Eating dinner too late or eating too little over the day—two classic setups for overeating at night.
2. Not budgeting out time to shop, so the cupboard is bare at dinnertime.

3. Too easily defaulting to eating out or ordering takeout. Especially if you live with someone, it's tough to be the one leading the charge to eat more meals at home, but readiness to change doesn't always occur simultaneously for people in a relationship. Be optimistic that if you lead, your partner will soon follow—or at least be supportive of your efforts.

Once you understand the carb-counting concept outlined in previous chapters, you can apply the strategies to just about anything you might contemplate eating. You can look at any recipe with a nutrition analysis listed and determine how much of it you can eat based on the carbohydrates per serving (and what you should or shouldn't eat with the entrée) and still stay within your carb budget. It's all about controlling the portions of the carb-containing parts of the meal. Let's go back to the balanced-plate idea:

Populate a quarter of your plate with protein. If you eat off a ten-inch plate (or smaller), a quarter of the plate should equal a roughly three- to four-ounce cooked portion of beef, pork, poultry, or seafood. To control calories, limit to occasional use (one a month or less often) foods that are fried or bathing in a cream sauce or heavy butter sauce. By all means, pan-fry in a small amount of oil (two tablespoons of oil used in a recipe that serves four is only 1^1/2 teaspoons of oil per person), or look for lighter versions of recipes in cooking magazines (my favorite is *Cooking Light*) or recipe websites. Otherwise, opt for grilled, baked, steamed, poached, or stewed meat, poultry, or seafood recipes.

Lean sources of protein include any kind of seafood, white meat poultry without the skin, and cuts of meat with the words "loin," "round," "flank," or 90 percent lean or leaner in the name. If you don't have a Crock-Pot, I encourage you to get one. What could be easier than putting all your ingredients for dinner in one pot in the morning and letting it cook all day while you're out? Layer chicken over a bed of cut vegetables, add some chicken broth, and season with your favorite herbs and spices. There are loads of Crock-Pot recipes on the Internet. Just be wary of high-fat ingredients.

Spice up your life. One challenge for many novice cooks is to figure out how to add flavor to recipes without adding too much fat. There's definitely trial and error involved, but the good news is that as American cuisine has gotten more multicultural, we've become more exposed to a greater variety of seasonings and spices. Culinary herbs and spices have been used medicinally for centuries. Beyond such traditional herbs as basil, oregano, dill, thyme, rosemary, and tarragon, there are countless herb and spice blends, like Italian and poultry seasonings, Asian spice mixes, and all kinds of "spicy" Southwestern and Indian blends for those who like a little kick to their food.

If you need some inspiration, one great resource for getting started is Penzey's Spices (www.penzeys.com), a mostly mail-order business that sells high-quality spices and provides hundreds of recipes on their website (and in their free catalog) explaining how to use them. Start simple by rubbing a new spice onto your chicken breast. You may be a more creative cook before you know it!

Get creative with your starch choice. Covering a quarter of your plate with a starch choice will help you avoid feeling deprived, but it should also be a reasonable enough portion to avoid spiking your demand for insulin. Higher-fiber grains are brown or wild rice, whole wheat pasta, alternative grains (like quinoa or barley), and whole grain bread. If you absolutely can't handle brown rice, opt for basmati white rice (which has a lower glycemic index than long grains). Colorful starchy vegetables are a super-healthy stand-in, providing both the carbs we crave and an assortment of healthy nutrients: sweet potato, yams, winter squash, corn, peas, and dried beans (kidney, garbanzo, pinto, and so on). Get creative and take low-carb vegetables—like carrots or string beans, for example—and make a gratin using reduced-fat cheese, where the bread-crumb-top crust is the starch but the bulk of the recipe is low-carb. If you're a vegetarian, combine the protein and starch parts of your plate. Here are some great ideas:

- Rice and beans
- Tofu, rice, and stir-fried vegetables
- Vegetarian chili and brown rice
- A veggie burger and a thirty-gram carb whole grain bun
- An egg, veggie sausage patty, and whole wheat English muffin sandwich

They're all plant protein plus starch combos. Beans, tofu, and textured vegetable protein (used to make veggie burgers and other meat substitutes) come packed with fiber, which helps mute their glycemic effect.

Salad for Supper: A Few Rules

Far too many people think that a salad consists of iceberg lettuce and salad dressing. Although iceberg lettuce has basically no calories and makes a nice filler, what you want from a salad are phytonutrients—plant chemicals that circulate around the body promoting good health. Many health-boosting phytochemicals also provide the pigment that gives plants their vivid colors, and iceberg lettuce has next to none. When you look at your salad, you should see color. Protein adds flavor and texture to a salad, and is absolutely necessary if you want it to be as filling as a meal. Try tossing in these ingredients:

- Grilled chicken
- Canned chicken or tuna
- Leftover meat, poultry, or seafood from last night's dinner
- Beans (kidney, garbanzo, black, pinto)—rinsed canned beans are fine
- Tofu cubes, soy nuts, edamame
- Reduced-fat cheese, shredded cheese
- Eggs and egg whites
- Small amount of strong-tasting cheese, like feta, blue, and Gorgonzola
- Nuts and seeds

A little healthy fat will add flavor and help you absorb the many fat-soluble phytonutrients in plant foods. Good sources of fat are nuts and seeds, avocado, olives, olive or canola oil, reduced-fat salad dressing, oil and vinegar, or a very small amount of full-fat dressing well tossed throughout the salad. Fresh or dried fruit can add flavor and texture to the salad. Try adding dried cranberries or raisins, mandarin orange slices, or chunked pineapple. You can almost feel how filling a salad with all of these ingredients would be. Pair it with a whole grain roll or pita and a glass of 1 percent or skim milk, and (voilà!) you have an incredibly nutritious, filling, and satisfying dinner.

Balanced-Plate Dinner Ideas

With all meal options, limit fat used in cooking to two tablespoons in a pan, and added fat at the table to two teaspoons (in the form of Smart Balance, Olivio, or other trans-fat-free tub spreads). It's okay to work in a teaspoon or two of butter here and there, but use butter sparingly: one tablespoon contains seven grams of saturated fat!

Balanced-Plate Dinner Ideas

DINNER CHOICE	CARBS (GRAMS)	
3–4 ounces cooked fish, poultry, or lean meat	0	
1 cup cooked sweet potato	30	**45 grams total** *(Note: It's okay to exempt the orange wedges from the carb count.)*
1 cup steamed asparagus	0	
Side spinach salad with almonds and mandarin oranges	0	
8 ounces skim or 1 percent milk	15	
2 teaspoons heart-healthy spread	0	
3–4 ounces grilled or stir-fried shrimp	0	
²/₃ cup brown rice or basmati rice	30	
1 cup steamed green beans with sesame seeds	0	**60 grams total**
8 ounces skim or 1 percent milk	15	
12 cherries	15	
2 teaspoons heart-healthy spread	0	
3–4 ounces chicken cacciatore	0	
Tomatoes, onions, peppers in the sauce	0	
1 cup whole wheat pasta	45	**45 grams total** *(Note: Be sure to measure out the whole wheat pasta—it's easy to go overboard!)*
Salad with greens, tomatoes, cucumbers, olives, and carrots	0	
1–2 tablespoons low-fat dressing	0	
Water or sugar-free beverage	0	
3–4 ounces sirloin steak or pork loin chop	0	
Half large baked potato	30	
Half cup steamed broccoli	0	**45 grams total** *(Note: Be sure to measure out the yogurt!)*
Half cup steamed carrots	0	
2 teaspoons heart-healthy spread	0	
Water or sugar-free beverage	0	
Half cup low-fat frozen yogurt	15	

Balanced-Plate Dinner Ideas, continued

DINNER CHOICE	CARBS (GRAMS)	
1 cup seasoned kidney or black beans, heated	30	
2/3 cup brown rice or basmati rice	30	
1 cup sautéed Brussels sprouts	0	60 grams total
Water or sugar-free beverage	0	
Sugar-free gelatin or frozen dessert ("0 carbs")	0	
2 cups salad greens	0	
Tomatoes, peppers, beets, olives, onions, carrots, artichokes, and quarter avocado	0	
3 ounces grilled or canned chicken	0	
Half cup garbanzo beans (chickpeas)	15	
2 tablespoons dried cranberries	15	60 grams total
1 tablespoon sunflower seeds	0	
Half Indian naan bread or one (six-inch) whole wheat pita	30	
2 teaspoons heart-healthy spread	0	
Water or sugar-free beverage	0	
1 tablespoon low-fat salad dressing	0	
One slice whole grain bread for half sandwich	15	
Two slices turkey, ham, or lean roast beef	0	
1 teaspoon light mayonnaise	0	
1 teaspoon honey mustard*	0	
1 cup tomato soup	15	45 grams total (*Free food because of the small portion.)
Salad with greens, grape tomatoes, cucumbers, peppers, and onions (or other vegetable on hand)	0	
2 tablespoons low-fat salad dressing	0	
5 chocolate candy pieces	15	
Water or sugar-free beverage	0	
2 cups of beef stew (made with lean beef, carrots, potatoes, and other vegetables)	30	
1 cup steamed broccoli	0	45 grams total
8 ounces skim or 1 percent milk	15	
Quarter (twelve-inch) pizza, cheese or veggie	30	
Large salad with at least five veggies and half cup kidney or garbanzo beans	15	
2 tablespoons low-fat salad dressing	0	60 grams total
Sugar-free fudge pop	15	
Water or sugar-free beverage	0	

Balanced-Plate Dinner Ideas, continued

DINNER CHOICE	CARBS (GRAMS)	
Three or four 1-ounce meatballs made with 90 percent lean ground beef	0	
1 cup whole wheat pasta	45	**60 grams total**
Tomato sauce	0	*(Again, measure the pasta. Also, use no-added-sugar or low-sugar tomato sauce.)*
1 cup steamed broccoli and cauliflower	0	
8 ounces skim or 1 percent milk	15	
1½ cups chili with ground turkey and beans	30	
⅓ cup brown rice	15	
2 tablespoons grated Parmesan cheese	0	**60 grams total**
1 cup steamed green beans	0	
8 ounces skim or 1 percent milk	15	
Sugar-free ice pop	0	
Two (six-inch) whole wheat tortillas	30	
3 ounces 90 percent lean ground beef or turkey breast, seasoned	0	
Half cup kidney or other dried beans	15	
Half cup part-skim grated Mexican cheese mix	0	
Shredded lettuce, diced tomatoes	0	**60 grams total**
One quarter cup salsa*	0	*(*Free in this amount.)*
1 tablespoon taco sauce*	0	
1 cup cantaloupe cubes	15	
Water or sugar-free beverage	0	

Keep in mind that even in these reasonable portions, the amount of fat you use in a recipe will strongly influence how many calories you consume. Mix and match your favorite foods now that you have a sense of carb-counting principles. Play around to find what works for you.

Boosting Your Intake of Plant Foods

Whether your goal is to control your PCOS, lose weight, follow the DASH diet (to lower your risk of diabetes, heart disease, and cancer), or all of the above, an important part of every health-promoting diet is to eat more plant-based foods. That's best accomplished by looking for ways to add fruits, vegetables, and unprocessed grains to each meal and snack whenever possible. The following tips may help you increase the odds of fitting these foods in:

- **Keep an open mind.** Fruits and vegetables you may not have liked earlier in life may be more appealing to you now. Start by trying new ones wherever you can—at a friend's house, at a party, in a restaurant, or at sampling stations at grocery stores.
- **Make time to shop.** Having these foods available in your home—and stored where you can see them—serve as reminders that you're trying to eat more plant-based foods. Keep fruit in a bowl on the kitchen table or counter (studies show people will eat more fruit if it's left in sight). Store vegetables on the refrigerator shelves where they're visible, as opposed to in the crisper bins, where you may forget about them.
- **Prep in advance.** When you get home from the store, immediately cut up fruits into fruit salad (try throwing in a can of pineapple chunks in water for a little added moisture), or prewash and chop fresh vegetables and store them in a resealable bag so all you have to do is pull them out and cook them at mealtime.
- **Cover half your plate.** Think of vegetables as something to eat at lunch and snack times as well as at dinner. At a meal cover half your plate with fruits and vegetables.
- **Fit some in by lunchtime.** Try to eat at least two servings of fruits and vegetables by lunch. It increases the odds you'll get in the recommended minimum of five to seven servings of fruits and vegetables by the end of the day. In general, a serving is half a cup cooked or one cup raw (or a piece of fruit about the size of a tennis ball).

There are dozens of simple ways to add fruits, vegetables, and whole grains to your meals and snacks. Start off by including a fruit with your breakfast. Try a sliced banana or berries in your hot or cold cereal, or some melon or an orange with your toast or eggs. Blend frozen fruit and plain yogurt to make a fruit smoothie. If you have more of a savory palate in the morning, add some sautéed vegetables—like onions, peppers, or broccoli—to scrambled eggs or an omelet. It's okay to count up to six ounces of 100 percent fruit juice as a fruit serving. Beyond that, however, opt for whole fruit.

Enjoy fruit as a midmorning snack. Put it out on your desk at work so you remember to eat it! Snack on yogurt with berries or dried fruit mixed in. Sliced fruit dipped in peanut butter or baby carrots dipped in hummus are other yummy options. For lunches and dinners, throw extra frozen vegetables into soups. Toss in rinsed canned beans to salads and canned soups for added protein and nutrients. At restaurants, choose soups with beans, or order veggie wraps, light on the dressing. Salad bars offer good opportunities to sample new vegetables.

For an easy meal to prepare at home, sauté beans (kidney, black, white, and pinto beans work well) in olive oil along with onions and garlic, then season with your favorite herbs or sauce, and serve with brown rice and other vegetables (such as steamed or sautéed broccoli, cauliflower, carrots, peppers, or zucchini). Throw cold leftover vegetables from the night before into a salad for lunch the next day. Add frozen vegetables (broccoli, cauliflower, carrots) to casseroles and tomato sauces to fill you up without an extra serving of pasta! Stuff a baked potato with canned diced tomatoes, peppers, onions, steamed broccoli, and reduced-fat grated cheese. Load up wrap sandwiches with greens, red peppers, and grated carrots.

· · ·

By this point I hope you've identified a few attractive options to get you started. Any meal component can easily be swapped out with any other option on the exchange lists for that food group (for example, swapping out a third cup of rice for a half cup of corn). The choice is up to you. It's often helpful to start with some basic meal ideas (like grilled chicken, brown rice, and steamed vegetables) where you can easily identify carbohydrates before moving on to combination meals where the carbohydrates may be less obvious (like chili, for example).

You're on your way to eating healthier, something that may have been on your list of things to do for a long time. But this time you know not just *what* to do with your diet, but *why* it makes a difference. You can visualize how making one food choice over another affects your blood sugar, insulin response, and appetite in a positive way. This knowledge makes all the difference in making your dietary changes stick. Understanding what's happening with your body and how what you eat affects it is empowering. Feeling physically and mentally better as a result may make it all worth the effort.

11

Mastering the Market: An Aisle-by-Aisle Shopping Guide

One of the greatest challenges for women with PCOS is planning meals and snacks so they're consistently making better food choices. It's one thing to know what you need to do, but making it happen is where the rubber meets the road. Step one toward healthier eating is to shop at the grocery store or farmers' market on a regular basis so you have what you need on hand. According to the Food Marketing Institute, in 2008 the average supermarket carried almost forty-seven thousand different items.[1] Once you pick up a box or package, the Nutrition Facts label contains an average of seventeen bits of data to look over, not counting any extended vitamin and mineral information the manufacturer may also decide to display.

Learning how to shop healthier is like any other new skill—with time and practice you'll learn how to replace your old grocery store choices with healthier alternatives. Initially, you should plan to spend more time wandering the aisles, reading labels, and finding substitutions for old favorites. Try not to see this as yet another unenjoyable task associated with a new "diet"; instead, this can be an empowering educational activity that's an important part of the journey toward lasting dietary change. Be patient. It takes time to transform your grocery cart into one full of healthy foods you'll enjoy eating. To make this learning process easier, I'll take you on an aisle-by-aisle supermarket tour, providing specifics on how to choose foods that are lower in fat and refined sugar and higher in dietary fiber and health-promoting nutrients.

Controlling Your Food Environment

There are few other investments in life that are as valuable as the contributions you make toward healthful eating. Never in our history has weight loss been the goal. Instead, our ingrained motivation has been to gain weight and store calories, so when we see or smell food, we want to eat it. How can we get past this natural human drive?

The solution is to control your food environment, which requires some advance planning and establishing a regular shopping habit. Populate the "up-close" spaces in your food environment with things you should be eating, and make it at least a little challenging to access those foods you may have trouble limiting. It's not about totally depriving yourself of foods you love. After all, food is one of life's great pleasures. If you want an ice cream, go out and get a child-size cone. That way you're not tempted every night by that half gallon of ice cream in the freezer. If you know you need an afternoon snack, pack one at home and bring it to work so it's easier to steer clear of the vending machine or the treats in the break room. Want to save calories and money? Pack a lunch from home, and make it the night before so you don't end up too busy to make it in the morning.

Controlling your food environment in these ways requires planning, a big part of which starts in the grocery store. Start by looking at your weekly schedule and decide where you'll fit in a trip to the store. Don't expect the time to shop to drop into your lap—plan for it like you would any other important weekly activity. Perhaps you'll do your shopping on Sunday evenings with a friend or family member, or maybe you'll hit the store on Friday afternoons, on your way home from work—scheduling a regular weekly hour or two for shopping is key. But once you're at the grocery store, how do you make good choices?

Reading Food Labels

The shopping lists in this chapter are organized by food category and begin with a brief description of what to look for on the label. Brand-name foods that meet the criteria are listed, but it's important to be able to navigate a food label yourself in case you find something that looks appealing and you want to know if it fits the bill. There are several things on the Nutrition Facts label that are most important to pay attention to.[2] Here's an example of a food label for multigrain bread.

Nutrition Facts

Serving Size 1 SLICE
Servings Per Container 20

Amount Per Serving

Calories 90	Calories from Fat 15

	% Daily Value*
Total Fat 2g	3%
Saturated Fat 0g	0%
Trans Fat 0g	
Cholesterol 0mg	0%
Sodium 130mg	5%
Total Carbohydrate 15g	5%
Dietary Fiber 2g	8%
Sugars 1g	
Protein 4g	

Vitamin A 0%	Vitamin C 0%
Calcium 4%	Iron 4%

Percent daily value reflects "as packaged" food.

* Percent daily values are based on a 2,000 calorie diet. Your daily values may be higher or lower depending on your calorie needs:

	Calories:	2,000	2,500
Total Fat	Less than	65g	80g
Sat Fat	Less than	20g	25g
Cholesterol	Less than	300mg	300mg
Sodium	Less than	2,400mg	2,400mg
Total Carbohydrate		300g	375g
Dietary Fiber		25g	30g

Calories per gram: Fat 9   Carbohydrate 4   Protein 4

Serving Size. The most important element on the food label is the serving size because everything else you subsequently read is based on that portion. If the label says a portion is a half cup and your portion is one cup, you need to double everything on the label. That's twice as many calories, fat grams, and carbs.

Calories and Calories from Fat. The next thing you see on the food label is "Calories" and "Calories from Fat." This is helpful information for determining whether the fat calories are a third or less of the total calories in the food item. One of the recommendations when following a heart-healthy diet is to eat foods that have roughly 30 percent or less of their calories from fat.

Total fat. This number helps you determine if a serving size of the food is "low-fat," which by definition means three grams of fat or less. Not all foods need to fit this definition, but it gives you a reference point for comparison. For example, something with five grams of fat is pretty close to low-fat, eight grams is getting up there, sixteen grams of fat in a hot dog is crazy!

Saturated fat and trans fats. These should be limited as much as possible in your diet, so ideally these two numbers on the food label should be zero. "Low saturated" means no more than a gram of saturated fat per serving, so aim for that with as many food choices as possible. Any amount of trans fat is considered unhealthy, so stick to that goal of zero. Keep in mind that if a nutrient is present in less than 0.5 gram per serving, the manufacturer is allowed to round down to zero on the label. This means there could be a hair less than 0.5 gram of trans fat per serving that could add up if you eat two or three servings. To play it safe, avoid foods with "shortening," "hydrogenated," or "partially hydrogenated" fat listed as an ingredient—these are the main sources of trans fats in the diet.

Cholesterol. "Low cholesterol" means no more than 20 milligrams per serving and should be limited to 300 milligrams a day.

Sodium. "Low sodium" means less than 140 milligrams per serving and should be limited to 2,400 milligrams a day (2,300 milligrams if you're following the DASH diet [Dietary Approaches to Stop Hypertension], mentioned in chapter 9).

Total carbohydrates. This number is of key interest to women with PCOS in managing their diet. A carbohydrate choice is a portion that contains fifteen grams of carb, so the total carb number should be divided by fifteen to see roughly how many "carb choices" are in a serving of the food. In the nutrition label above, the fifteen grams of carb a serving of this food is one choice.

Dietary fiber. This is an important part of the PCOS diet plan as well. The more fiber you eat the better. A high-fiber food means there's five grams or more per serving. A food that is considered a "good source" of fiber has 2.5 to 4.9 grams per serving. Remember, with any food that contains five grams of fiber or more per serving, you are allowed to subtract half the grams of fiber from the total carbs in your carb count. For example, if total carbs are twenty-five grams per serving and dietary fiber is six grams, you "count" the food as having twenty-two grams of carbohydrate per serving.

Sugar. There is currently no official definition for "low sugar," because food labels don't differentiate between natural sugars (fructose from fruit and lactose from milk) and added sweeteners. "Reduced sugar" means 25 percent less sugar than the original, which doesn't necessarily mean much if the original is loaded with sugar. A reasonable number to aim for is around eight grams of sugar or less per serving. When thinking in terms for the day, aim for a limit of twenty-five grams of added sugar total for the day (the same as saying a hundred calories from added sugars per day), not including "sugars" from fruit and milk, which are natural.

Protein. The presence of protein in a carb-containing food will help you feel fuller longer and slow the digestion of carbs to blood glucose.

Percent Daily Value. This is the amount of a nutrient that will be satisfied by eating one serving of the food item. The percents are based on the levels of nutrients recommended as part of a healthy two-thousand-calorie diet as listed at the bottom of the Nutrition Facts label. In the figure above, a serving of our sample food will use up only 5 percent of the sodium allowance for the day (listed at the bottom of the label as 2,400 milligrams). Percent Daily Values are also provided for some vitamins and minerals. Worth noting is that the calcium percentage is based on the daily value of 1,000 milligrams; if you replace the percent sign with a "0," that equates to your milligrams. In the figure above, the 4 percent calcium daily value represents 40 milligrams of calcium.

Eating Plant Foods:
Aim for a Combination of Colors

An important part of the PCOS diet plan is to eat more plant foods. Varying the color palette of your fruits and vegetables will assure a variety of nutrients in your diet much more effectively than any vitamin pill you can pop. Many of the healthful nutrients found in plant foods (the phytonutrients) give them their color. Check out this color-coded list of fruits and vegetables, and make it a goal to stretch beyond your old standbys:

- **Blue/purple.** Blueberries, blackberries, eggplant, figs, plums, prunes, purple cabbage, and purple grapes.

- **Green.** Artichokes, arugula, asparagus, avocado, bok choy, broccoli, broccoli rabe, Brussels sprouts, cabbage, celery, cucumbers, endive, greens, green apples, green beans, green grapes, green olives, green peppers, honeydew melon, kiwi, limes, lettuce, okra, peas, snow peas, spinach, and zucchini.
- **Orange/yellow.** Apricots, cantaloupe, carrots, corn, grapefruit, lemons, mangoes, nectarines, oranges, papaya, peaches, pineapples, pumpkin, sweet potato, summer squash, tangerines, winter squash, yams, yellow beets, and yellow pears.
- **Red.** Beets, cherries, cranberries, pink grapefruit, pomegranates, radishes, radicchio, raspberries, red apples, red grapes, red onions, red peppers, strawberries, tomatoes, and watermelon.
- **White/gold.** Bosc pears, cauliflower, garlic, jicama, mushrooms, onions, parsnips, potatoes, shallots, and turnips.

When buying produce, aim for fresh as often as possible, but also stock up on frozen vegetables so you have a backup when you've run out of fresh veggies. I'm a huge fan of steam-ready microwavable vegetables. Frozen vegetables are steamed right in the bag like microwave popcorn, and according to the companies, all the plastics used are FDA-approved as microwave safe. For those who prefer to avoid cooking in plastic, you can cook fresh or frozen veggies in a stainless-steel vegetable steamer. Frozen fruits are also nice to have on hand to mix with yogurt (if you thaw the fruit slightly first) or blend into a smoothie.

Many of my patients are interested in whether they should be eating organic. This question remains unresolved due to lack of data on the long-term health of people who have long eaten organic. One thing is certain: hundreds, if not thousands, of studies support the benefits of eating more plant foods regardless of how the fruits and vegetables are grown. Cost is certainly a factor for some people as well in the decision between conventional and organic produce. While the science continues to evolve, those interested in "going organic" may want to start with the "Dirty Dozen," a list compiled by the Environmental Working Group that identifies the twelve most pesticide-contaminated fruits and vegetables that may be worth spending precious organic food dollars on. The "Dirty Dozen," from most to least contaminated, are celery, peaches, strawberries, apples, blueberries, nectarines, bell peppers, spinach, kale/collard greens, cherries, potatoes, and grapes (imported). You can download a list of the "Dirty Dozen" (and the "Clean Fifteen," the least-contaminated fruits and vegetables) at www.foodnews.org/walletguide.php.

Starter Shopping List

Now that you know how to read labels and have a sense that portions matter most, let's take a look at a shopping list that can help guide you through the supermarket aisles. These lists are by no means meant to be all-inclusive. Criteria are provided at the top of each category that you can apply to anything of interest. Examples of foods that meet the criteria are here to get you started. Most items included here are readily available, but you may need to visit a health-food store to find a few depending on where you live. Also keep in mind that product lines do sometimes change over time. Start experimenting and see what you can add to—or what you should subtract from—your kitchen!

Poultry. Note that "Cold cuts" are listed separately, later in the shopping list.

- Canned chicken: for sandwiches and salads (mix with low-fat mayo or dressing)
- Chicken legs and thighs: fresh or frozen, remove the skin to cut fat calories
- Fresh chicken breast: buy in bulk when on sale and freeze individually in freezer bags
- Fresh or frozen turkey breast
- Frozen chicken breast: available in large resealable plastic bags as breast or tenders, or individually frozen in plastic
- Ground turkey that is 90 percent lean or leaner
- Limit chicken wings, nuggets, and any other breaded product to only occasional use due to high fat (and salt) content
- Precooked chicken pieces: beware the sodium in flavored varieties

Seafood. Buy fresh, frozen, or canned depending on use.
- Any kind of fresh or frozen fish or seafood that's not fried
- Canned tuna or salmon

- Salmon lox
- Smoked salmon

Meat. Look for the words "loin," "round," "flank," "chuck," or 90 percent lean or leaner. Limit your meat intake to no more than eighteen ounces a week.[3]
- Beef: eye of the round, top round steak, top round roast, sirloin steak, top loin steak, tenderloin steak, and chuck arm pot roast
- Lamb: leg, loin chop, and arm chop
- Pork: tenderloin, top loin roast, top loin chop, center loin chop, sirloin roast, loin rib chop, and shoulder blade steak
- Veal: cutlet, blade or arm steak, rib roast and rib, or loin chop

Miscellaneous protein. The following are great choices for vegetarians, or anyone interested in incorporating more plant proteins into their diet.
- Beans (black beans, chickpeas, kidney beans, and so on) and peas
- Eggs and egg substitutes
- Soy foods: tofu, tempeh, textured vegetable protein (TVP)
- Veggie burgers and other soy-based meat alternatives

Fats and oils. Focus on heart-healthy fats; avoid products with trans fats. Remember: All fats are equal in calories, regardless of how heart-healthy (or not) they are.
- Light mayonnaise
- Low-fat salad dressings (these generally taste better than fat-free dressings, but be sure to watch your portions)
- Nut butters (there is no need to buy reduced-fat peanut butter—just watch your portions)
- Nuts and seeds
- Olive, canola, or peanut oil
- Olives
- Tub spreads: trans-fat-free (such as Olivio, Smart Balance, Brummel & Brown, Promise, many "light" spreads)

Cereals. Look for cereals with at least three, preferably five or more, grams of fiber, and no more than eight grams of sugar per serving. If your favorite cereal is higher in sugar, try mixing a quarter cup of it with three-quarters of a cup of low-sugar, high-fiber flakes—that way you get a taste of your favorite with a dose of added fiber!

- Barbara's cereals: Cinnamon Puffins (not Peanut Butter Puffs), Original Puffins, Multigrain Shredded Spoonfuls, and Shredded Wheat
- Cascadian Farm cereals: Pomegranate Raspberry Clusters, Cinnamon Crunch, Clifford Crunch, Purely O's, and Hearty Morning
- General Mills cereals: Cheerios (other flavored versions of Cheerios, including Honey Nut, Apple, and Berry, have only 2 grams of fiber per serving), Fiber One, Fiber One Honey Clusters, Multibran Chex, Multigrain Cheerios, Total Whole Grain, Wheaties, and Wheat Chex
- Health Valley cereals: Amaranth Flakes, Oat Bran Flakes, and Organic Fiber 7 Multigrain Flakes
- Kashi: Autumn Wheat (mini wheats), Go Lean, Good Friends, Heart to Heart Honey Toasted Oat, Mighty Bites Honey Crunch, and 7 Whole Grain Flakes
- Kellogg's cereals: Complete Oat Bran Flakes, Complete Wheat Bran Flakes, All Bran, and Special K low carb
- Post cereals: Bran Flakes, 100% Bran, Grape Nut Flakes, Shredded Wheat, and Shredded Wheat and Bran
- Quaker cereals: Corn Bran, Oatmeal (preferably plain Old Fashioned, which cooks quickly in microwave; if buying flavored oatmeal, opt for the "lower sugar" instant option)
- Trader Joe's and Whole Foods grocery stores: Both nationwide stores carry many varieties that meet these criteria; read the labels carefully.

Crackers. Look for low-fat crackers (no more than three grams of fat), with two grams of fiber or more, and no trans fats.
- Ak-mak 100% Whole Wheat
- Graham Crackers (any brand)
- Kashi TLC Honey Sesame; Kashi TLC Natural Ranch
- Kavli whole grain crisp breads
- Reduced Fat Triscuits

- Reduced Fat Wheat Thins; Wheat Thins Harvest Five Grain; Wheat Thins Crisps
- Wasa Multigrain
- Whole Foods "365" brand Baked Woven Wheats

Bread products. Breads, bagels, English muffins, and other bread products should say "whole grain" as the first ingredient on the label whenever possible, and contain at least two to three grams of fiber per slice. Opt for breads with seventy to ninety calories per slice.

- Breads with two grams of fiber per slice: Arnold Health Nut, Arnold Stone Ground 100% Whole Wheat, Canadian 100% Whole Wheat, Cape Cod 100% Whole Wheat, Gold Medal 100% Whole Wheat, JJ Nissen Canadian-Style Multigrain, Martin's Whole Wheat Potato Bread, Matthew's Whole Wheat, and Wonder Stone Ground 100% Whole Wheat
- Breads with three grams of fiber per slice: Arnold Branola Natural Whole Grain (the "original" bread), Bouyea Fassetts Stone Ground 100% Whole Wheat, Pepperidge Farm Crunchy Grains Natural Whole Grain, Pepperidge Farm Dark Wheat Natural Whole Grain, Pepperidge Farm 9 Grain Natural Whole Grain
- Bagels: Thomas's New York Style Bagels (with ten grams of fiber), whole grain mini bagels
- Other: Joseph's Oatbran & Whole Wheat Tortilla wrap (six grams of fiber each), Food for Life: Bran for Life bread (five grams of fiber per slice, available frozen at Whole Foods)

Cold cuts. Look for low-fat varieties (three grams fat per serving), although cold cuts may still be high in sodium and should be limited.

- Beef: extra-lean roast beef
- Ham: Plumrose 99 percent fat-free cooked (0.5 fat gram per slice), Lean Cuisine ham slices, Carl Buddig baked honey ham (extra lean), Healthy Choice Ham (97 percent fat-free), Oscar Meyer 96 percent fat-free ham (smoked)—three slices contain 1.5 grams of fat and 790 milligrams of sodium!
- Turkey: Oscar Meyer turkey breast, Healthy Choice 97 percent fat-free turkey, Louis Rich fat-free turkey breast, Carl Buddig lean

turkey, Butterball fat-free chicken and turkey breast slices, Hebrew National oven roasted turkey breast (99 percent fat-free)

Cheeses. Look for cheeses with five grams of fat or less per ounce or slice. These are made with fat-free, low-fat, or part-skim milk. Some cheeses listed here have slightly more fat, but they are still good choices when eaten in moderation.

- American: Smart Beat, Kraft-free singles, Borden fat-free singles, Kraft 2 percent milk singles, Land-O-Lake light
- Cheddar: Cabot 50 percent milk Deli Deluxe, Cracker Barrel 2 percent milk (six grams of fat), Laughing Cow Mini Babybell Mild, Sargento Medium or Sharp Deli style thin, Sargento Reduced Fat Sharp Cheddar Sticks
- Feta: President fat-free feta, Alpine Lace reduced-fat feta, Organic Valley feta, Trader Joe's Authentic Greek feta, Stella feta, Athenos reduced-fat feta, Athenos mild feta
- String cheese: Borden Double Twist, Borden part-skim mozzarella, Polly-O Stringums part-skim mozzarella (six grams of fat), Polly-O Twistums mozzarella and cheddar (four grams of fat), Sargento's Twirl (five grams of fat), Sorrento's Stringsters part-skim (five grams of fat), Trader Joe's part-skim mozzarella
- Swiss cheese: Laughing Cow Light Creamy Swiss Original, Jarlsberg light, Sargento reduced-fat deli-style thin, Kraft 2 percent milk Deli Deluxe, Finlandia Heavenly light

Yogurts. Unless it's plain (unflavored), yogurt may contain large amounts of sugar unless marked "light," which means the item has been artificially sweetened. Look for 1 percent or nonfat varieties.

- Chobani nonfat Greek yogurt
- Columbo Light
- Dannon Light & Fit, Dannon fat-free plain yogurt
- Fage nonfat Greek yogurt
- Other 1 percent or nonfat Greek yogurts
- Stonyfield Farm (plain or flavored) or Oikos Greek
- Yoplait Light

Milk. Milk should be skim or 1 percent milkfat as 2 percent is very close in fat content to whole milk.

- Any skim or 1 percent milk
- Over-the-Moon: 1 percent fat or fat-free (both have the taste of whole milk)
- Lactaid-brand fat-free or 1 percent milk (for those with lactose intolerance)
- Silk soy milk, Silk soy milk (enhanced) with 35 percent Daily Recommended Value for calcium, 8th Continent-brand vanilla soy milk (with one gram of fat), Nature's Promise soy milk (with 3.5 grams of fat)
- Simply Smart: nonfat milk with the taste of 2 percent milk

Beverages. All beverages should have no more than forty calories per eight-ounce serving.

- All diet soda waters, seltzer waters
- Apple and Eve Light and Fruitful Cranberry, Cranberry, Raspberry
- Arizona Diet Green Tea, Nestle Diet Iced Tea
- Crystal Light
- Diet Snapple beverages
- Diet V-8 Splash
- Fruit 2O
- Light Ocean Spray Crangrape, Cranberry, Cranraspberry
- Minute Maid Light juice beverages
- Vitamin Water 10 (sweetened with Stevia), Smart Water

Frozen foods. Some frozen foods may be low in calories and fat, but many are still very high in sodium. Look for frozen dinners with forty-five to sixty grams of carb, at least ten grams of protein, no more than eight to ten grams of fat, and no more than 500 milligrams of sodium whenever possible. Add extra fresh or frozen vegetables to boost the plant content of the meal.

- Frozen foods: natural food stores offer healthier frozen dinners (try such brands as Amy's, Organic Bistro, Kashi, and others)
- Vegetarian alternatives: Garden Burgers (meatless, soy-based); Boca Products (meatless, soy-based); meatless "chicken patties," meatless chili, soy breakfast patties; Morningstar Farms burgers, sausages,

and other products; Nature's Promise soy veggie burger; soy "crumbles" from either Morningstar Farms or Green Giant, Dr. Praeger's meatless burgers and other meatless products

Snack foods. Look for low-fat options, meaning three grams of fat or less per serving. Many are carbs that should be paired with protein for a more filling snack. Limit these foods to one serving a day, preferably less.

- Chips: Baked Lay's potato chips, Cape Cod 40 percent reduced-fat potato chips, Genisoy Crisps, Glenny's Soy Crisps, Ruffles Light Fat Free Potato Chips, Tortilla Chips, Doritos Light Tortilla Chips, Guiltless Gourmet Baked Tortilla Chips, Baked Tostitos
- Miscellaneous: Pepperidge Farm Snack Sticks, Stella D'oro breadsticks, Nature Valley Crunchy Granola Bars, Nature Valley Chewy Trail Mix Bar, Nature's Promise Granola Bars, Quaker Chewy Granola Bars (not chocolate covered), Uncle Sam's Cereal Bars (oatmeal raisin), Kashi TLC Honey Almond Flax Chewy Granola Bars, Kashi TLC Chewy, Crunchy, and Fruit & Grain granola bars, Nature Valley Fruit & Nut Bars, Quaker Mini or regular Rice cakes (plain or flavored), Quaker Corn cakes (plain or flavored)
- Pretzels: any plain pretzel (get unsalted when used for dipping), Rold Gold Plain or flavored pretzels, Rold Gold Braid Honey Wheat Pretzels, Snyder's of Hanover (any kind except Sourdough Hard Honey, Mustard, and Onion pieces—these are high in fat)
- Popcorn: Light Microwave Popcorn (trans-fat-free), Boston Lite Popcorn (50 percent less fat), Newman's Own 94 percent Fat Free Butter, Orville Redenbacher's Light Butter, Pop Secret 94 percent Fat Free Butter
- Pudding snacks: Hunt's Fat Free Snack Pack Pudding or Tapioca, Jell-O Gelatin cups (regular or sugar-free), Mott's Healthy Harvest Applesauce cups, or other "natural" (no-sugar-added) applesauce

Sweets. Look for cookies with no trans fats (be careful: some will have zero trans fats per serving but still some hydrogenated fat that could add up). Limit these foods to one serving a day, preferably less, to control your calories. And remember to factor in the carbs!

- Low-fat frozen desserts: Limit these to one serving to control calories. Remember to factor in the carbs.
- Products with artificial sweeteners: Welch's No Sugar Added Fruit Juice Bars, Original Fudge Bar No Sugar Added, Hood Simply Slender Mini ice cream sandwiches, Klondike Slim-a-Bear Bars No Sugar Added, The Skinny Cow No Added Sugar ice cream sandwiches
- Products without artificial sweeteners: Hendries Citrus Six, Edy's whole fruit bars, Luigi's Real Italian Ice, Silhouette Low Fat ice cream sandwich, Skinny Cow ice cream sandwiches

There you have it. Some basic guidelines, aisle-by-aisle, to master the market. Although retooling your shopping habits may seem overwhelming at first, there are a few things you can do to make it more interesting and efficient:

1. **Shop with a partner or friend.** Getting support around healthy eating from those closest to you greatly increases your odds of success. These people may also offer you a few helpful ideas.

2. **Shake up your shopping destinations.** Visiting different specialty markets where food is often displayed in an appealing way may jog your culinary interest. Local farm stands or produce markets may even offer samples of fruits and vegetables to taste-test. Be adventurous and try something new! You never know what you might discover.

3. **Be prepared.** Preparing even just part of a meal in bulk can really lighten the cooking load during the week. Maybe grill up a bunch of chicken on the weekends to eat hot or cold at meals during the week. Then all you have to do is prepare some vegetables or a starch to be served on the side.

· · ·

The bottom line for mastering the market is to think ahead. Plan *when* you're going to do your shopping and *what* you'd like to eat. You don't need to change everything at once. You might start with just one meal. Focus on better breakfast choices, healthy foods to pack and bring into the office for lunch, or redefining dinner. Just keep moving ahead!

12

Negotiating the Menu: Dining Out

It certainly may be healthier to plan and prepare a wholesome meal at home every night, but in today's on-the-go society that's not always possible. Is it possible to control your food environment when eating out? Yes! You *can* dine out and still eat healthfully. Nutrition is a hot topic today, and most restaurants will offer at least a few healthy options, even if the portions are larger than they should be. With a little strategic planning—and some guidance on how to make special requests—you should be able to walk into almost any eating establishment confident that you can find something to fit your needs.

Part of the reason it may be so hard for many of us to resist overeating when dining out is that we may still experience that "yippee!" feeling we had as kids, when eating out was a special treat. As one of six siblings, I didn't go out to eat very often as a child. When we did, it was definitely a moment to celebrate. We ordered all kinds of foods that we didn't usually have at home. The problem for many of us as adults is that dining out has become a lifestyle habit where that old "yippee" mind-set can get us into trouble!

As Americans have become accustomed to eating out more often, restaurants have sought to cater to every taste and price point to claim a piece of the dining-out pie. It's easier to make decent choices at some types of restaurants than at others, but most make it tough to control your portions. Fast-food restaurants—like McDonald's, Burger King, Wendy's, and KFC—make it nearly impossible unless you order a kid's meal, which technically should also be enough for the average adult. Not far behind are chain restaurants—like T.G.I. Friday's, Applebee's, Chili's, and the Cheesecake Factory—where, although they may offer a calorie-controlled item, the rest of the menu is loaded with highly processed, tough-to-resist foods that are high in fat, salt, and sugar. Of course it is all delivered in enormous portions. Your best bet is to dine at smaller restaurants, where the food is prepared on site and it's easier to get an idea of what's actually in the meal.

Regardless of where you're dining out, start with two basic assumptions:

1. The portion is probably at least 30 to 50 percent larger than you should be eating (unless you're a marathon runner!).
2. The amount of fat and salt (and sugar) in the meal is probably a lot higher than you think.

If you're really determined to eat a healthy meal, try to request substitutions (an extra vegetable instead of french fries, for example) and modifications in the preparation (sauce on the side, less butter, and so on). With the rising rates of food allergies in our society and an increasing focus on health, many restaurants are used to being asked what's in their food and if something can be served differently.

Even if you find a restaurant with reasonably healthy options, the portion sizes will likely present a challenge. These strategies will help you deal with this difficult reality:

- Split a large entrée with someone else. You'll save both cash and calories.
- Ask the server to pack up half your entrée in a take-home container before you're even served.
- Some restaurants have lighter-fare items on the menu that are either smaller portions or made with lower-calorie ingredients—these would be the smarter choice.
- Avoid all-you-can-eat buffets! Very few people can resist the temptation to overeat in these food-sensory-overload settings. Why make it so hard on yourself?

Navigating the Menu

Dining out is a fact of life, so learning how to spot healthier options is a critical skill, particularly if you travel for work and eat out frequently. These guidelines will help you navigate each part of the plate to make lower fat and calorie choices.

Meat, poultry, and seafood. When ordering these items, foods described with these words imply cooking methods that are high in fat and calories: "fried," "crispy," "pan-fried," "parmesana," "sautéed," and "stuffed." Instead, look for these words that suggest a much lighter method of cooking: "steamed," "broiled," "baked," "grilled," "poached," and "roasted." Fatty cuts of meat include rib eye, porterhouse, and T-bone. Leaner cuts are London broil, filet mignon, round or flank steak, sirloin tip, and tenderloin. If you're not sure how a certain dish is prepared, ask your server. Request any visible fat to be removed from the meat and the skin to be removed from poultry before it's served. Request that gravies, sauces, and dressings be served on the side, so you can control how much you eat (don't use it all!), or skip these often high-calorie additions completely.

Starches and vegetables (side dishes). High-fat side starch and vegetable dishes are often described on menus with these words: "fried," "scalloped," "au gratin," "in a cream or cheese sauce," and "tempura-style" (fried vegetables). When choosing entrées, look for choices that are served with a lot of vegetables. Steer clear of creamy sauces and other high-fat methods of preparation. Remember the balanced-plate approach: cover half the plate with vegetables by trading in the starch for a second vegetable. You can then savor a roll with butter as your starch. Look for plain vegetables that are steamed, grilled, or roasted; ask for a lemon wedge to add flavor.

When choosing from starchy sides, try to order whole grains like brown or wild rice, whole wheat tortillas, and whole wheat pasta when possible (these items might be difficult to find in many restaurants). Higher-fat starch choices include rice pilaf, stuffed or "twice baked" potatoes, and vegetable or potato casseroles. A reasonable portion of rice (choose brown rice if it's available) or half a baked potato are better options than these. It can be easy to go overboard with butter and sour cream: keep in mind that every teaspoon of butter you melt over the top of a potato adds 40 calories, and a measly two tablespoons of sour cream adds 50 calories.

Other Helpful Hints

- Limit yourself to one piece of bread or skip it altogether if one slice is likely to lead to many. Avoid fatty breads like croissants and gooey rolls and pastries.
- Experiment with ethnic foods, which often use unique spices and fresh herb blends to season the cuisine and rely less on salt and fat. The same principles apply, however: if you don't know what's in it, ask; be on the lookout for fried and other high-fat foods; curb your carb intake; and search the menu for extra vegetables.

Salad. Salad with low-fat dressing can be a great premeal filler, making it easier to not overindulge on the main entrée. To conserve calories, ask for dressing on the side and dip your fork into it before grabbing a bite of salad. Just because it has the word "salad" in it doesn't mean it's healthy, but salads can be smart choices with a little attention to the ingredients. Salad bar add-ons that can undo the health value of a salad are mayonnaise-based pasta and potato salads, oil-based marinated vegetable or bean salads, cheeses, croutons, and bacon bits. If you can't resist lacing your salad with a small amount of these fatty add-ons, conserve on calories by limiting yourself to a modest amount of low-fat dressing. Choose a low-fat vinaigrette over a creamy dressing. It's thinner, which makes it easier to spread around and use less. Love blue cheese dressing? Mix a teaspoon of it with two tablespoons of low-fat Italian for a little blue cheese flavor without the calories! Because it's drenched with dressing, caesar salad is usually loaded with fat and calories. The only way to salvage this situation is to order the dressing on the side and use sparingly. A Greek salad that's overflowing with feta cheese and olives is also loaded with fat and calories. The remedy? Ask for half the cheese, limit yourself to five olives, and use a low-fat dressing.

Pizza. If you order pizza, try to find someone (or two!) to split it with, and choose healthier toppings like spinach, mushrooms, broccoli, and roasted peppers. Always order a salad with low-fat dressing to additionally fill you up first, so you can limit yourself to a slice or two of pizza. Avoid deep dish, stuffed crust, and all other manner of super-fattening pizza (this means limiting the meat toppings).

Pasta. Choose tomato-based marinara or primavera sauces rather than cream-based sauces. Tomato sauce delivers a fraction of the calories of cream sauce and actually counts as a vegetable serving! Be brave and ask for half the plate to be covered with the vegetable of the day. Halving your plate of pasta will halve your carbs for the meal. Try covering the veggies with tomato sauce to trick your brain into thinking you've had a full plate of pasta.

Soups. Broth-based soups are low in calories and make a great premeal filler. Or they can be part of a calorie-controlled entrée when paired with a salad. Creamed soups, bisques, and chowders are much higher in calories. Limit these choices to special occasions.

Seafood. Fish and seafood dishes are great if you order them baked, broiled, poached, steamed, grilled, or lightly sautéed. Although it is delicious, deep-frying seafood may add unhealthy saturated fats and can more than double the calories. And above all, try to resist the side order of fries. Instead, ask for extra vegetables.

Vegetarian entrées. These can be great choices if they're not loaded with butter, cheese, and fried vegetables. Vegetarian entrées are more likely to include whole grains, beans, and other high-fiber foods. Be adventurous and try tofu. It takes on the flavor of whatever it's cooked in, so you might be pleasantly surprised.

Hamburgers. This is a tough one. To make the most of it, order the smallest burger on the menu (or try a turkey or veggie burger). Other tips: watch the amount of cheese and mayo, eat only half the bun, and ask for a salad to replace the giant side order of french fries that almost universally comes with burgers. A regular fast-food restaurant hamburger (about the size of what you'd find in a children's meal) is about three hundred calories, ten to fifteen grams of fat, and thirty-five grams of carbohydrate.

Mexican food. Right off the bat, ask your server not to bring the requisite basket of fried tortilla chips to the table. On the menu look for whole wheat tortillas, beans, and grilled entrées. Steer clear of deep-fried entrées (like chimichangas) and dishes with loads of cheese and sour cream. If you order a taco salad, don't eat the fried shell.

Dessert. Although it may be tough to look beyond the chocolate cake and ice cream sundaes, some restaurants offer sorbet (which is fat-free) or fresh fruit as dessert options. If you decide to go for your favorite delectable treat, however, ask someone to split it with you. You might also suggest a dessert that the whole table can share.

Beverages. Beverages can add an overwhelming number of calories to a meal if you're not careful. The 250 calories from a twenty-ounce soda or 150-calorie beer can tally up quickly. In place of soda or other sweetened beverages, choose water, diet soda, seltzer water with lemon or lime, low-fat milk, tea, or coffee. If you're consuming alcoholic beverages, limit them to one drink a day or less. One alcoholic drink is a twelve-ounce beer, fives ounces of wine, or $1^1/2$ ounces of spirits.

Talking to Your Server

If you frequent many of the same restaurants, talk to the wait staff, manager, or chef to get their advice on which menu items meet your needs and preferences. If you don't know how something is prepared, by all means, ask. Don't be afraid to request that an entrée be prepared with less fat or salt, or to make substitutions to lower the carb or calorie content of a meal. Restaurants are part of the hospitality industry—they want you to come back. Most chefs will go above and beyond to please.

If you find yourself often in search of healthy meal options in the various places you travel, try searching your locations in advance at www .healthydiningfinder.com. This website compiles dietitian-approved menu items from restaurants throughout the country. Simply plug in your zip code and see who offers healthy choices in your area. The search results include the nutrition breakdown for the items offered. A great book on the ins and outs of healthful dining is *Eat Out, Eat Right* by diabetes expert Hope Warshaw.[1] This handy little book walks you through every kind of cuisine imaginable, offering insights on what to choose and what to avoid.

．．．

Although dining out is a modern-day fact of life, making healthful choices in the face of all the sensory temptations restaurants exude can be a real challenge. Even if you order a healthier option, the portion may be twice what you should eat. Limiting your exposure to these tough-to-navigate situations by eating out less often is a good place to start. But armed with some background nutritional know-how—and determination to ask for what you need—you can still enjoy a guilt-free evening out, confident that your PCOS diet plan is still on track.

PART 4

PCOS and Other Considerations

13

Finding Support and Relieving Stress

Now that we've discussed the integral role of diet and exercise in managing PCOS, it's time to look beyond those aspects of the PCOS diet plan to address the emotional challenges this condition presents. The other key part of managing the condition is lining up the support that can help you see through the confusing and overwhelming times. When you're diagnosed with a condition that many people haven't even heard of, finding a team to help you develop—and stick with—a health plan can be invaluable. You're particularly lucky if you have access to a PCOS support group—who could better understand what you're dealing with than others with the same issues? In lieu of that, a health-care provider, behavioral health therapist, mind-body practitioner, partner, friend, or other health-focused group can also provide the support needed to manage both your physical and emotional health as it relates to PCOS.

Without question, having PCOS can wreak havoc on your emotional health for a number of reasons:

- Lifelong struggles with weight loss that seem fruitless.
- A sense of lack of control over what's happening with your body.
- Fear of chronic health problems, like diabetes and heart disease.
- The already emotionally charged challenges of infertility.
- Body image issues related to obesity, excess hair growth or hair loss, and skin problems.
- Disordered eating (particularly compulsive eating and bulimia).
- Not being understood or taken seriously by health-care professionals, family, or friends.

Scientific research supports the reality that having PCOS indeed presents some unique emotional challenges. A review of major articles published between 1985 and 2009 dealing with the psychological aspects of the syndrome found that depression and other emotional stressors frequently negatively affected emotional well-being, self-image, and quality of life. Major sources of stress are hirsutism, obesity, irregular periods, and problems with fertility, with obesity being the most prevalent cause of emotional distress for women with PCOS.[1]

One study on incidence of depression compared 103 women with PCOS to 103 women without the condition and found depressive disorders in 21 percent of the women with PCOS, compared with only 3 percent of those without it. Compared with the nondepressed PCOS women, the depressed PCOS women had a higher Body Mass Index (BMI) and more evidence of insulin resistance.[2] Research looking specifically at quality of life reached a similar conclusion, with women with the condition reporting lower quality-of-life scores than women without PCOS, with BMI again being a significant player. On the positive side, the researchers found that providing these women with good-quality information on managing their PCOS improved quality-of-life scores.[3]

Diet, Mood, and Emotional Health

Whether a woman has PCOS or not, we know that how we eat can affect our mood and emotional health. A recent study looking at the dietary patterns of almost thirty-five hundred middle-age men and women found that those whose diets were heavily loaded with fruits, vegetables, and fish had a lower risk of depression than those who ate a highly processed diet of sweetened desserts, fried food, processed meats, refined grains, and high-fat dairy products.[4] Other preliminary research has suggested a tie between elevated androgen levels, food cravings, and mood problems. All of this research points to the value of controlling PCOS for both physical and emotional health reasons.[5]

As with most overweight women, body image concerns are a major issue for women with the condition. Add some facial hair, thinning hair on the crown of the head, and a sense that your body just isn't doing what it's supposed to and you have a recipe for body dissatisfaction. It appears that exercise is one of the most positive things you can do to improve how

you feel about your body. Some research has found that even without leading to a significant change in BMI, moderate exercise can help women feel
better about themselves, improving their quality of life.[6] Countless times
I've heard women report how much better they feel, physically and emotionally, by adding even modest amounts of activity to their life. Exercise
helps ease depression and anxiety in a number of ways:

- It increases production of "feel-good" neurotransmitters and endor-
  phins (those responsible for that talked-about "runner's high").
- It blunts the release of immune system chemicals that can aggravate
  depression.
- It increases body temperature, which can have a calming effect.
- It provides a socially appropriate means of working off negative
  energy.
- It removes chemical by-products of the body's fight-or-flight stress
  response by simulating the fight-or-run activity that is supposed to
  be fed by this reaction, thereby helping the body recover from this
  instinctive stress response quicker.
- It helps increase self-confidence in what you think your body is
  capable of (often much more than you think!).
- It gets you in touch with your muscles from the neck down, which
  may improve self-esteem and how you feel about your appearance.
- It distracts you from what's troubling you, potentially short-circuiting
  a cycle of negative thoughts.
- It may help provide structure to your day, which for many people is
  comforting.

People who are anxious or depressed may also feel socially isolated, and
exercise gets them out in the world. If you go to a gym or exercise class at
the same time often enough, you may start to connect with other people
who have similar goals. Even better is identifying a supportive exercise
buddy—invite a friend to meet you regularly for an exercise class or a walk
around the neighborhood. For many people not exercising itself is a source
of stress, because you know you should but aren't. Getting up and moving
can help relieve the anxiety that you're not taking care of yourself.

De-Stressing with Mind-Body Therapies

Beyond establishing a regular exercise routine, the mind-body world offers many alternative therapies that can help you feel relaxed and give you a chance to appreciate what it means to feel good. Indulging in massage therapy, acupuncture, Reiki, qigong, aromatherapy (use of essential oils from plants to support and balance the mind, body, and spirit), meditation, prayer, art, music, and dance, to name a few activities, may be helpful to include in a physical and emotional health improvement plan.

Most people are familiar with acupuncture, which uses very fine needles inserted into specific points on the body for therapeutic purposes. Acupuncture is a form of traditional Chinese medicine that is based on the concept that disease results from disruption in the flow of qi (vital energy) and imbalance in the forces of yin and yang, and aims to restore and maintain health through the stimulation of specific points on the body. Many of my patients find acupuncture very relaxing (many of whom are receiving acupuncture for fertility-related purposes), and, despite the use of needles, I've never heard it described as painful. Reiki is a healing practice that originated in Japan. Reiki practitioners place their hands lightly on or just above the person receiving treatment, with the goal of facilitating the person's own healing response.[7] Qigong, an ancient practice for manipulating one's own qi to benefit one's physical, emotional, mental, or spiritual health, incorporates stress-reduction techniques including regulated breathing, visual imagery, meditation, and various gentle movements.[8]

Some strategies—like listening to music, practicing meditation, using aromatherapy, and regular citations of prayer—are inexpensive or free. They're also easy to access at any time. In my practice I've heard many women sing the praises of massage and acupuncture for relaxation—although these therapies are more expensive, particularly if used on a regular basis, a fortunate few may have some health insurance coverage for massage and acupuncture, so check your plan. I've had less experience with Reiki and qigong in women with PCOS, but in general these therapies can be very helpful as a means of relaxation (and exercise in the case of qigong). They are also useful therapies for visualizing your path to good health. You may need not look any further than your community adult education programs to find an outlet for art or dance. Try something new to get creative, get moving, and get de-stressed. Whatever your budget allows, be sure to carve out time to take care of this aspect of your health.

When to Ask for Help

When dealing with PCOS, it's also important to know when you need more than self-help. Beyond diet, nutrition, and stress-relieving techniques, take stock of the kinds of support you need for managing the syndrome. Don't be afraid to ask for help. Stress is often not something outside yourself that you find threatening, but rather, it is your *response* to that thing. Finding a way to change how you respond to stress is a vital part of feeling more in control of your life. Support groups can be a fantastic way to establish a network so you don't feel alone in your struggles. Many women in infertility support groups may also be dealing with PCOS, so local fertility treatment centers may be a good resource if you're grappling with that issue. If you're comfortable with the idea of online support, online communities (like www.pcosupport.org, www.soulcysters .com, and www.pcoschallenge.com) are there twenty-four hours a day to lend a hand.

If weight loss is part of your plan, consider joining Weight Watchers (www.weightwatchers.com to find a local chapter), TOPS (Take Pounds Off Sensibly, www.tops.org to find a local chapter), or some other community or fitness organization–based weight-loss support organization. Find a supportive doctor to work with. If your gynecologist doesn't specialize in PCOS, ask for a referral to a reproductive endocrinologist who does. Look for a registered dietitian (RD) in your area who specializes in treating PCOS to help you change your eating habits and lose weight. The American Dietetic Association's "Find a Registered Dietitian" link at www.eatright.org can connect you with RDs in your area.

You may need a therapist to help you manage stress or deal with some long-standing personal or behavioral issues that the PCOS diagnosis may have brought to the forefront. Don't be afraid to reach out for this kind of support. Many of our most self-destructive or tough-to-control habits have been reinforced for years, and they may take a long time to rewire. Unhealthful coping mechanisms you may have come to rely on—like binge eating, stress eating, or finding excuses to avoid exercise—may benefit from the input of a trained mental health professional, particularly if disordered eating or severe depression are present. A thorough discussion of managing eating disorders is beyond the scope of this book. But if binge eating and purging or any other out-of-control eating behaviors are present, a team therapy approach (including a physician, therapist, and registered dietitian) is critical for recovery. Find someone to work with to help you untangle what's been going on and how to change it. It's not a weakness to admit you need help. It actually shows strength to admit you can't go it alone. I've worked with some incredible therapists in my professional life and have great respect for the role they play in helping to get people moving forward. Referrals to licensed behavioral health professionals can be found through your primary care doctor, health insurance plan, or employee assistance program.

. . .

Managing PCOS and all that goes with it is stressful! It takes a lot of emotional energy to make major lifestyle changes. The fear of what you think this diagnosis may mean to your overall health can be paralyzing. It can be particularly overwhelming if you're also struggling with infertility. But help is out there. Sometimes getting support for what's emotionally weighing you down is what opens the door to the possibility of changing unhealthful diet and lifestyle habits that have been holding you back for years. Whether you simply start exercising to blow off steam, delve into self-help strategies, or enlist the help of a mental health professional, now is the time to rally all the support necessary to get your health under control.

14

PCOS and Planning for Pregnancy

By far, the best thing you can do to set the stage for a healthy pregnancy is to manage your PCOS. Obesity presents a fertility problem whether you have PCOS or not, so if weight is an issue for you, losing weight will help align your hormones and increase your odds of conceiving. Losing weight will also reduce your risk of developing gestational diabetes when you do get pregnant. Obesity is also a known risk factor for neural tube defects, fetal mortality, and preterm delivery. Even if you're not overweight, the guidelines outlined here can help manage any underlying insulin resistance to maximize your odds of conception. In a perfect world all women with PCOS would know they have the condition and therefore have a chance to work on diet and lifestyle change *before* they try to conceive. Unfortunately, many women aren't diagnosed with PCOS until they've tried to get pregnant without success and end up seeing a reproductive endocrinologist. This can be particularly true of women who have a variant of PCOS, where they do get their period but still have hormonal issues that may be interfering with conception. As if the infertility thing wasn't stressful enough, now you may feel pressure to shift into high gear on a diet and exercise plan, which can be even more stressful if you feel that your biological clock is ticking loudly.

Research on Nutrition and Pregnancy

According to a position paper on nutrition and pregnancy from the American Dietetic Association, the quality of a woman's diet heading into a pregnancy matters. Despite this, studies show that many women in the

United States don't consume a healthy diet before, during, and after pregnancy. According to the Dietary Guidelines for Americans, many adult women may not be getting sufficient amounts of calcium, fiber, magnesium, vitamins A and C, potassium, and carotenoids (a raw material for vitamin A).[1] What's more, 30 to 40 percent of women consume inadequate levels of vitamins A, C, B6, and folate, and iron deficiency is relatively common, which is particularly troublesome considering both iron and folate play critical roles in conception and fetal development.[2]

As many as 50 percent of pregnant women, and upwards of 60 percent of breast-fed babies, are believed deficient in vitamin D despite widespread use of prenatal vitamins. The 400 IUs of vitamin D in many prenatal vitamins is thought to be too low to promote healthy blood levels (30 nanograms per milliliter or higher) in many pregnant women and breastfeeding infants. Taking 400 IUs of vitamin D in addition to a regular multivitamin or prenatal multi may help most women achieve sufficient levels of vitamin D in the body. Low levels of vitamin D are associated with preeclampsia (a dangerous late-pregnancy condition marked by high blood pressure and protein in the urine), low infant weight, and other newborn health problems. New recommendations for vitamin D intake are expected in 2010.[3] (For more details on the importance of vitamin D intake for women with PCOS generally, see chapter 8.)

Preconception Nutrition:
Ten Healthy Pre-Pregnancy Steps

Beyond managing insulin resistance and weight, planning for pregnancy for women with PCOS is the same as it would be for any woman contemplating pregnancy. The idea is to send the strongest message possible that the body is healthy enough to be pregnant, and the odds of successful reproduction are good. In the months leading up to a pregnancy, there are some simple steps you can take to stock up on a few essential nutrients, clear the decks of anything potentially toxic to pregnancy, and make sure any underlying heath problems are as well controlled as possible.

Any woman contemplating pregnancy should start priming her body for the healthiest pregnancy possible. According to my conversations with nutritionist Elizabeth Ward, author of *Expect the Best: Your Guide to Healthy Eating Before, During, and After Pregnancy*: "Before you try for a baby, you should address any issues you might have with weight; have a complete physical exam that includes tests for glucose and iron; curb your use of anything potentially unsafe for pregnancy; and start eating healthfully, including supplementing with any nutrients you need to have the healthiest baby possible."[4] Whether you should try to lose weight and get healthier before you attempt to conceive should be discussed with your physician, who will take into account your whole clinical picture, including your age. If you have the luxury of time, however, developing a diet and exercise plan to improve the quality of your diet and manage insulin resistance can enhance your odds of a healthy pregnancy for both you and your baby.

There are many things you can do during preconception to hedge your bets for a healthy experience. Below are ten preconception steps toward a healthy pregnancy.

1. **Evaluate your weight.** Being over- or underweight can hinder your attempts at conception. If possible, aim for a Body Mass Index (BMI) in the healthy range, ideally between 20 and 24.9. If a BMI below 25 seems difficult, don't despair. Research shows that even modest weight loss can improve fertility in women with PCOS.[5] Being underweight can also make it more difficult to conceive, so reach for a minimum BMI of 20.

2. **Move it.** Research shows that regular exercise is necessary for weight loss, and is a vital part of an overall health improvement plan. Exercise is also one of the most natural ways to short-circuit any stress you might be experiencing. Set a goal of thirty to sixty minutes of moderate-intensity activity most days. Walking will do just fine. If you're in treatment for infertility, you may want to tone down vigorous exercise to moderate levels to avoid overheating your body.

3. **Take a multivitamin.** All women of childbearing age should take a multivitamin containing 400 micrograms of folic acid to decrease the risk of neural tube defects (although sometimes doctors prescribe larger doses of folic acid if there is a personal or family history of neural tube defects).[6]

4. **Beef up your blood.** Iron is important for reproduction, so get a test for iron deficiency anemia. Take iron supplements if recommended by your doctor, and increase your food sources of iron, like meat,

poultry, seafood, iron-fortified cereals (look for those with 45 percent of the recommended daily value or higher), beans, tofu, and spinach. Take foods and supplements with a source of vitamin C (citrus fruits and juice, tomatoes, potatoes, peppers, broccoli, and strawberries) to enhance iron absorption.

5. **Increase your D.** In addition to your multivitamin (or prenatal vitamin if recommended by your doctor), take an additional 400 IUs of vitamin D for a total of at least 800 IUs from supplements. If you are taking a calcium supplement, it may contain vitamin D as well, which counts toward this total. Any additional vitamin D from milk and other vitamin D–fortified foods is a bonus.

6. **Stock up on DHA.** If you don't eat twelve ounces a week of fatty fish such as salmon, bluefish, mackerel, herring, sardines, and lake trout, take a DHA (docosaohexaenoic acid) supplement or fish oil supplement providing at least 200 micrograms of DHA for your baby's brain and retinal development.[7] Women stockpile DHA better when body fat stores are low, so the preconception phase is a great time to start. Avoid eating fish high in mercury—swordfish, shark, king mackerel, and tilefish. Low-mercury fish and shellfish include shrimp, salmon, pollack, canned light tuna, and catfish. Limit albacore, or white tuna, to six ounces a week, as it has more mercury than light tuna.

7. **Abstain from substances unsafe for pregnancy.** Stop smoking, avoid alcohol, set aside herbal supplements, and review any prescription and over-the-counter medications with your doctor so you know what's safe to take during pregnancy.

Metformin and Pregnancy

If you do get pregnant and have been taking the insulin-sensitizing medication metformin, don't be surprised if your obstetrician or reproductive endocrinologist recommends keeping you on the medication for a while (or for the duration of your pregnancy). Some physicians are now using this strategy as a means of possibly reducing the risk of miscarriage and gestational diabetes.[8] Discuss your specific situation with your doctor.

8. **Curb your caffeine.** The March of Dimes recommends that women who are pregnant or trying to become pregnant limit their caffeine intake to 200 milligrams a day, which is about the equivalent of sixteen ounces of regular coffee or four cups of tea. But numbers do vary by brand. For example, that "small" sixteen-ounce coffee at Starbucks contains about 320 milligrams of caffeine. Caffeine may increase the risk of miscarriage in some women.[9] If you're undergoing in-vitro fertilization (IVF) you may want to limit caffeine even further. One study of 221 couples undergoing IVF suggests a potential benefit to limiting caffeine to less than 50 milligrams per day (approximately the amount in eight ounces of tea or four ounces of regular coffee). Although there's no scientific consensus on this issue, it can't hurt to play it safe.[10]

9. **If you have diabetes, know your numbers.** Blood glucose levels need to be normal, or as close to normal as possible; there is serious risk of birth defects if the fetus is exposed to excess blood glucose in the first trimester.[11]

10. **Become familiar with pregnancy weight gain recommendations.** Studies suggest up to 43 percent of women gain too much weight during pregnancy.[12] Gaining too little is also unhealthy for both you and your baby. New recommendations on this from the Institute of Medicine are as follows:
    - Underweight (BMI is less than 18.5):
      total weight gain range is twenty-eight to forty pounds.
    - Normal weight (BMI between 18.5 and 24.9):
      total weight gain range is twenty-five to thirty-five pounds.
    - Overweight (BMI between 25.0 and 29.9):
      total weight gain range is fifteen to twenty-five pounds.
    - Obese (BMI greater than 30.0):
      total weight gain range is eleven to twenty pounds.[13]

. . .

Even though PCOS can present some unique conception and pregnancy challenges, I see women with PCOS become pregnant and have babies all the time. If you've had trouble getting pregnant, the single most important thing you can do is to get any underlying insulin resistance under control so that you're ovulating more consistently. Even if you do get your period every month, keep in mind the influence of insulin can be subtle, so it's possible to have very mild insulin resistance that you would benefit from controlling. Following the PCOS diet plan and practicing the strategies in this book may positively influence your cycle and enhance your pregnancy odds. It's a well-balanced plan that's healthy for a number of reasons. These preconception suggestions—supplementing with folic acid, DHA, and iron, if necessary; watching your weight and overall health; exercising moderately; and ridding your diet of unhealthy substances—will not only prepare you for the healthiest pregnancy possible but help you feel better physically and emotionally regardless of pregnancy plans. Preconception time also presents a great opportunity to practice some mind-body techniques you may find incredibly valuable in the months to come (see chapter 13 for some wonderful mind-body therapies).

15

Integrating the PCOS Diet Plan into Your Life

So there you have it: a detailed plan to help you manage polycystic ovary syndrome through diet and lifestyle change. Having PCOS may be the best excuse in the world for you to finally work on changing any unhealthy habits and routines. This book makes the case for *why* what you do with food, activity, and lifestyle choices makes a difference, especially if you're dealing with PCOS. Here are a few reminders:

- **Healthy food choices.** Your food choices can either aggravate your insulin resistance or improve it.
- **Exercise.** Physical activity is "natural medicine" for insulin resistance and is essential for both weight loss and stress management.
- **Supplements.** Sensible dietary supplementation can optimize the nutrient profile of your diet for better health, and maybe even help manage your mood.
- **Self-care.** Tending to your emotional needs is essential to your overall health and can make picking a plan and sticking with it more achievable.

Much of what people read about diet and nutrition is confusing. They want to eat better but they don't really know how, which can become yet another source of stress. Many people have an all-or-nothing view: if you can't change radically all at once, why bother changing at all? But research tells us this is not how people alter their habits for the long term. The slow-and-steady approach is more effective, because it generally means you're doing the hard work of looking at your diet and lifestyle habits one at a time and brainstorming ways to adjust them in a permanent way. Being realistic about how long it will take to change those habits is important.

Remember: This is a process, not an event. Only crash diets for weight loss make false promises about amazing changes happening overnight and achieving painless transformations. Your path may be tediously slow— addressing one habit, meal, or task at a time. Or maybe you've decided you're ready to go, and you move along at a steady, determined pace. This is often particularly true of women who are highly motivated to get pregnant and time is of the essence.

Clearly, there will be challenges along the way. They could be situational: Perhaps you live with someone who has been your eating buddy and now you're ready to change but he or she isn't. Or you work very long days and are challenged to find time to fit in exercise or meal planning. Your obstacles could be emotional: Perhaps you have a long-standing habit of self-medicating stress and sadness with food, or you don't have any confidence that you're even capable of change. It could also be that you're *just not ready*. In my experience readiness for change can make all the difference in whether someone can pick up the ball and run with it or feel stuck. I hope that reading *The PCOS Diet Plan* has moved you a little closer to readiness. If so, consider even this small step progress.

Like any health problem, there will always be uncertainties in managing your PCOS. Regardless of your efforts, you may still struggle with infertility or health complications from the condition. But without question, eating better, increasing your activity, and developing stress-relieving strategies will improve your quality of life. You'll experience a sense of empowerment, like you're not just waiting for doctors to make you feel better—*you* are doing it! You're pitching in, taking charge, and hedging your bets that trying something new is better than doing nothing at all. Whatever path (or pace) works for you in learning to manage your PCOS is fine. It's *your* story—*you* get to write it. My hope is that *The PCOS Diet Plan* has provided you with the necessary tools to succeed in your journey toward improved health.

Apendix 1:
Sample Meal Plans

Below are four varied-calorie meal plans (1,400, 1,600, 1,800, and 2,000) to help you figure out how to distribute your carbohydrates and calories over the course of the day. They are designed to be a blueprint to get you started, and can be fine-tuned to your preferences as you begin to get a handle on the carbohydrate-distributed diet. Here are several things to consider and keep in mind as you develop your personalized plan:

- People who lose weight and keep it off tend to eat in a structured manner that helps them stay ahead of their hunger and on track with your goals. This approach greatly enhances the odds you'll be successful on the carbohydrate-distributed diet plan as well.
- You may find the 1,400-calorie meal plan quite restrictive. It's best to get serious about the exercise piece so you have a little more food flexibility.
- These meal plans do not factor in any small portions of "free foods" you might incorporate into meals and snacks.
- As long as there is reasonable balance in where your carbohydrates are coming from, it's possible to trade carbs from a starch for a serving of dairy, for example, or a fruit serving for a starch serving, so that you have some day-to-day flexibility in what you're eating but the carbohydrate dose is roughly the same.
- If you want to factor in a small portion of dessert you need to trade in some carbs, preferably from the starch and dairy group so that you can maintain your daily fruit intake of at least two fruits.
- Not every day goes perfectly. These meal plans are designed to guide how you eat 80 to 90 percent of the time. This represents your habits. The occasional transgression is expected as part of "normal eating." What matters is that you prioritize getting right back on track.

1,400-Calorie Meal Plan (45 to 60 grams of carb per meal, 15 grams of carb per snack)

BREAKFAST	GRAMS OF CARB
2 Starch	30
1 Protein	0
1 Dairy	15
1 Fruit	15
1 Fat	0
SNACK	
1 Fruit	15
LUNCH	
1 Starch	15
2 Protein	0
1 or more Nonstarchy vegetables	free
1 Dairy	15
1 Fat	0
SNACK	
1 Starch	15
1 Protein	0
DINNER	
2 Starch	30
2 Protein	0
2 or more Nonstarchy vegetables	free
2 Fats	0
1,414 calories	**82 grams protein (23 percent)**
159 grams carb (45 percent)	**50 grams fat (32 percent)**

1,600-Calorie Meal Plan (45 to 60 grams of carb per meal, 15 grams of carb per snack)

BREAKFAST	GRAMS OF CARB
2 Starch	30
1 Protein	0
1 Dairy	15
1 Fruit	15
1 to 2 Fats	0
SNACK	
1 Fruit	15

1,600-Calorie Meal Plan, continued

LUNCH	
1 Starch	15
3 Protein	0
1 or more Nonstarchy vegetables	free
1 Dairy	15
1 Fat	0
SNACK	
1 Starch	15
1 Protein	0
DINNER	
2 Starch	30
3 Protein	0
2 or more Nonstarchy vegetables	free
2 Fats	0
1,644 calories	**96 grams protein (23 percent)**
185 grams carb (46 percent)	**56 grams fat (31 percent)**

1,800-Calorie Meal Plan (45 to 60 grams of carb per meal, 15 grams of carb per snack)

BREAKFAST	GRAMS OF CARB
2 Starch	30
1 Protein	0
1 Dairy	15
1 Fruit	15
1 to 2 Fats	0
SNACK	
1 Fruit	15
LUNCH	
2 Starch	30
3 Protein	0
1 or more Nonstarchy vegetables	free
1 Dairy	15
1 Fat	0
SNACK	
1 Starch	15
1 Protein	0

1,800-Calorie Meal Plan, continued

DINNER	
2 Starch	30
4 Protein	0
2 or more Nonstarchy vegetables	free
1 Dairy	15
1 Fruit	15
2 Fats	0
1,827 calories	**114 grams protein (25 percent)**
201 grams carb (44 percent)	**65 grams fat (31 percent)**

2,000-Calorie Meal Plan (45 to 60 grams of carb per meal, 15 grams of carb per snack)

BREAKFAST	GRAMS OF CARB
2 Starch	30
1 Protein	0
1 Dairy	15
1 Fruit	15
1 to 2 Fats	0
SNACK	
1 Fruit	15
LUNCH	
2 Starch	30
3 Protein	0
1 or more Nonstarchy vegetables	free
1 Dairy	15
1 Fruit	15
1 Fat	0
SNACK	
1 Starch	15
1 Protein	0
DINNER	
3 Starch	45
4 Protein	0
2 or more Nonstarchy vegetables	free
1 Dairy	15
2 Fats	0
1,998 calories	**117 grams protein (24 percent)**
216 grams carb (43 percent)	**74 grams fat (33 percent)**

Appendix 2: Food Journal

Keeping a food journal is a scientifically proven way to stay attuned to how you're eating and help you stick with your goals. Try making a commitment to track the times you eat or drink, what you had, how much, the grams of carb per portion and how hungry you were on a scale of 1 to 10 (1 being "not hungry," 10 being "starved"). Remember, eating when your hunger is a 5 or 6 increases the odds of being able to control your portions.

DATE/ TIME	FOOD/BEVERAGE CONSUMED	AMOUNT EATEN	GRAMS OF CARBS	HUNGER SCALE (1–10)

Resources

The following websites are helpful if you're looking for more information about PCOS and its related issues.

Polycystic Ovary Syndrome

National Women's Health Information Center, U.S. Department of Health and Human Services
www.womenshealth.gov/faq/polycystic-ovary-syndrome.cfm
The U.S. Department of Health and Human Services women's health website answers frequently asked questions about PCOS.

SoulCysters
www.soulcysters.com
The largest online community of women with PCOS.

Polycystic Ovarian Syndrome Association, Inc.
www.pcosupport.org
Formed in 1987, PCOSupport is an all-volunteer grassroots organization that is operated by women with PCOS and those who support them.

Center for Young Women's Health, Children's Hospital Boston
www.youngwomenshealth.org/pcosinfo.html
A PCOS website for teens from Children's Hospital, Boston, Massachusetts.

PCOS Challenge: The Support System to Help Women Beat PCOS
www.pcoschallenge.org
The PCOS Challenge is a program that brings women with PCOS together to support each other in managing their PCOS.

OBGYN.net PCOS Pavilion
www.obgyn.net/pcos/pcos.asp
OBGYN.net PCOS Pavilion is a physician-reviewed site offering medical professionals and women the latest news and information on Polycystic Ovary Syndrome.

Pregnancy

Expect the Best Pregnancy
www.expectthebestpregnancy.com
Website and blog of Elizabeth Ward, MS, RD, author of *Expect the Best: Your Guide to Healthy Eating Before, During, and After Pregnancy*.

The March of Dimes
www.marchofdimes.com
Website of the March of Dimes, the leading nonprofit organization for pregnancy and
baby health.

Mindful Eating and Eating Disorders

The Center for Mindful Eating
www.tcme.org
The Center for Mindful Eating (TCME) outlines the principles of mindful eating and
resources available to help implement them.

Mindless Eating
www.mindlesseating.org
Website of Brian Wansink, PhD, author of *Mindless Eating: Why We Eat More Than
We Think.*

National Eating Disorders Association
www.nationaleatingdisorders.org
The NEDA website provides support for people and families affected by eating disorders.

National Institute of Mental Health
www.nimh.nih.gov/health/publications/eating-disorders/complete-index.shtml
Webpage on eating disorders. Describes the different types of eating disorders, symptoms, and treatments.

General Nutrition and Healthy Eating

American Dietetic Association
www.eatright.org
The public section of this website provides extensive food and nutrition resources for
consumers.

Fruits & Veggies, More Matters
www.fruitsandveggiesmorematters.org
A great resource to learn more about the benefits and nutritional value of fruits and
vegetables. Gives menu ideas to incorporate more fruits and veggies for a family on a
budget. Full of practical tips.

Harvard School of Public Health
www.hsph.harvard.edu/nutritionsource
The Nutrition Source explores the latest science about healthy eating for adults,
answering key questions and providing practical tips for increasing the overall quality
of your diet. Includes tips and recipes for eating more fruits and vegetables.

MyPyramid
www.mypyramid.gov
MyPyramid offers personalized eating plans and interactive tools to help you plan
and assess your food choices based on the Dietary Guidelines for Americans. The
MyFood-A-Pedia tool provides quick food lookup and food comparisons.

Center for Science in the Public Interest
www.cspinet.org
Website of the *Nutrition Action Healthletter*, an award-winning website ideal for keeping up on what is happening in the field of nutrition and health.

Dietary Guidelines for Americans 2010
www.cnpp.usda.gov/DGAs2010-DGACReport.htm
Provides detailed information on the USDA's Dietary Guidelines for Americans and
how to implement them.

Useful Tools for Tracking Food, Activity, and Goals

Nutrition Facts and Calorie Counter
www.nutritiondata.com
Provides complete nutrition information for foods and helps you select foods that best
match your dietary needs.

Calorie King
www.calorieking.com
Very comprehensive, useful website with a food database containing the nutritional
information for most American generic and brand-name foods (including the common fast-food chains).

FitDay
www.fitday.com
Provides a free account including an online diet journal for tracking food, exercise,
weight loss, and health goals. Includes a diet analysis tool to view your daily calories,
nutrition, and weight-loss progress.

The Daily Plate
www.thedailyplate.com
Free online food diary and activity tracker. Database includes almost 700,000 foods
and 1,500 activities along with helpful calculators to set and track weight, activity,
and diet goals. Includes nutrition information for many restaurant chains.

Sparkpeople Online Weight-Loss and Fitness Support
www.sparkpeople.com
Offers free diet and fitness plans, calorie and exercise trackers, fitness videos, and other
tools, along with a supportive online community.

Reference Websites

Consumer Lab
www.consumerlab.com
Excellent resource for deciding on a quality dietary supplement or herbal products. Tests and reviews a variety of supplements, reports their findings on the supplement's content and quality, and then rates them as approved or disapproved for use. Small annual fee required in order to log into website.

Memorial Sloan-Kettering Cancer Center
www.mskcc.org/mskcc/html/11570.cfm
Free herb and dietary supplement database from the Integrative Medicine Service of New York's Memorial Sloan-Kettering Cancer Center. Provides evidence-based information about herbs, botanicals, supplements, and more.

Glycemic Index
www.glycemicindex.com
Official website of the glycemic index and Glycemic Index/Glycemic Load database.

Healthy Cooking

Cooking Light
www.cookinglight.com
Website of the highly respected *Cooking Light* magazine that provides thousands of free recipes tested by their staff of professionals and registered dietitians to meet stringent nutritional requirements and high flavor standards.

EatingWell
www.eatingwell.com
Website of *Eating Well* magazine that provides thousands of beautifully presented, healthful recipes.

Epicurious
www.epicurious.com/recipesmenus/healthy/recipes
Healthy recipes section of Epicurious.com, a website dedicated to recipes, cooking, drinking, entertaining, and restaurants.

The World's Healthiest Foods
www.whfoods.com
This website designed for the real "foodie" offers extensive information on the benefits of eating healthy foods, along with a comprehensive database describing the nutritional benefits of hundreds of foods and how to select, store, and prepare them (also includes scientific study citations to support information).

Notes

Introduction

1. Samuel Thatcher, *PCOS: The Hidden Epidemic* (Indianapolis, Ind.: Perspectives Press, 2000).

Chapter 1

1. Helen Mason, "Polycystic Ovary Syndrome (PCOS) Trilogy: A Translation and Clinical Review," *Clinical Endocrinology* 69, no. 6 (2008): 831–44. David Ehrmann, "Medical Progress: Polycystic Ovary Syndrome," *New England Journal of Medicine* 352 (2005): 1223–36.

2. David Ehrmann, "Medical Progress: Polycystic Ovary Syndrome," *New England Journal of Medicine* 352 (2005): 1223–36.

3. Ibid.

4. Elbert Huang, "Projecting the Future Diabetes Population Size and Related Costs for the U.S.," *Diabetes Care* 32, no. 12 (December 2009): 2225–29.

5. "Polycystic Ovary Syndrome: Frequently Asked Questions," available online at www.womenshealth.gov/faq/polycystic-ovary-syndrome.cfm#k.

6. David Ehrmann, "Medical Progress: Polycystic Ovary Syndrome," *New England Journal of Medicine* 352 (2005): 1223–36.

7. Samuel Thatcher, *PCOS: The Hidden Epidemic* (Indianapolis, Ind.: Perspectives Press, 2000).

8. Tasoula Tsilchorozidou, "The Pathophysiology of Polycystic Ovary Syndrome," *Clinical Endocrinology* 60, no. 1 (2004):1–17.

9. P. Crosignani, "Polycystic Ovarian Disease: Heritability and Heterogeneity," *Human Reproductive Update* 7, no. 1 (2001): 3–7.

10. Julian Barth, "The Diagnosis of Polycystic Ovary Syndrome: The Criteria Are Insufficiently Robust for Clinical Research," *Clinical Endocrinology* 67, no. 6 (2007): 811–15.

11. On the use of insulin-sensitizing agents, see "Practice Committee of the American Society for Reproductive Medicine. 2009. Use of Insulin-Sensitizing Agents in the Treatment of Polycystic Ovary Syndrome," *Fertility & Sterility* 90 (S3): S69–S73. On the use of metformin, see S. Palomba, A. Falbo, F. Zullo, F. Orio Jr., "Evidence-based and Potential Benefits of Metformin in the Polycystic Ovary Syndrome: A Comprehensive Review," *Endocrine Reviews* 30, no. 1 (2009): 1–50; ACOG Committee on Practice Bulletins—Gynecology, "ACOG Practice Bulletin No. 108: Polycystic Ovary Syndrome," *Obstetrics & Gynecology* 4 (2009): 936–49; K. Hoeger, K. Davidson, L. Kochman, T. Cherry, L. Kopin, and D. S. Guzick, "The Impact of Metformin, Oral Contraceptives, and Lifestyle Modification on Polycystic Ovary Syndrome in Obese Adolescent Women in Two Randomized, Placebo-Controlled Clinical Trials," *Journal of Clinical Endocrinology & Metabolism* 11 (2008): 4299–306; and R. J. Norman, R. Dewailly, R. S. Legro, and T. E. Hickey, "Polycystic Ovary Syndrome," *Lancet* 370, no. 9588 (2007): 685–97.

12. American Heart Association, "Third Report of the National Cholesterol Education Program (NCEP) Expert Panel on Detection, Evaluation, and Treatment of High Blood Cholesterol in Adults (Adult Treatment Panel III): Final Report," *Circulation* 106 (2002): 3143–3421.

13. R. Azziz, "Position Statement: Criteria for Defining Polycystic Ovary Syndrome as a Predominantly Hyperandrogenic Syndrome: An Androgen Excess Society Guideline," *Journal of Clinical Endocrinology and Metabolism* 91, no. 11 (2006): 4237–45.

Chapter 2

1. C. Archard and J. Theirs, "Le virilsme pilaire et son association a l'insuffisance glucolytique (diabetes des femmes a barb)," *Bulletin of the Academy of National Medicine* 86 (1921): 51–64.

2. J. Chang, "Insulin Resistance in Non-Obese Patients with Polycystic Ovarian Disease," *Journal of Clinical Endocrinology and Metabolism* (1983). A. Dunaif, "Profound Peripheral Insulin Resistance, Independent of Obesity, in Polycystic Ovary Syndrome," *Diabetes* 38 (1989): 1165–1174.

3. T. Tsilchorozidou, "Pathophysiology of Polycystic Ovary Syndrome," *Clinical Endocrinology* 60, no. 1 (2004): 1–17.

4. "Insulin Resistance and Prediabetes," National Diabetes Information Clearing House, available online at http://diabetes.niddk.nih.gov/DM/pubs/insulinresistance/.

5. Eric Westman, "Is Dietary Carbohydrate Essential for Human Health?" *American Journal of Clinical Nutrition* 75, no. 5 (May 2002): 951–53.

6. "Diabetes Fact Sheet," Centers for Disease Control, 2007, available online at www.cdc.gov/diabetes/pubs/pdf/ndfs_2007.pdf.

7. Gerald Reaven, "The Metabolic Syndrome: Is a Diagnosis Necessary?" *American Journal of Clinical Nutrition* 84, no. 5 (November 2006): 1253.

8. Tasoula Tsilchorozidou, "The Pathophysiology of Polycystic Ovary Syndrome," *Clinical Endocrinology* 60, no. 1 (2004): 1–17. David Ehrmann, "Medical Progress: Polycystic Ovary Syndrome," *New England Journal of Medicine* 352 (2005): 1223–36.

9. Tasoula Tsilchorozidou, "The Pathophysiology of Polycystic Ovary Syndrome," *Clinical Endocrinology* 60, no. 1 (2004): 1–17.

10. International Diabetes Federation, "Consensus Worldwide Definition of the Metabolic Syndrome," available online at www.idf.org/webdata/docs/IDF_Meta_def_final.pdf.

11. Sven Benson, "Maladaptive Coping with Illness in Women with Polycystic Ovary Syndrome," *Journal of Obstetric, Gynecologic, and Neonatal Nursing* 39, no. 1 (January 2010): 37–45.

Chapter 3

1. S. E. Kasim-Karakas, "Relation of Nutrient and Hormones in Polycystic Ovary Syndrome," *American Journal of Clinical Nutrition* 85, no. 3 (March 2007): 688–94.

2. S. E. Kasim-Karakas, "Effects of Protein versus Simple Sugar Intake on Weight Loss in Polycystic Ovary Syndrome," *Fertility and Sterility* 92, no. 1 (July 2009): 262–70.

3. K. Stamets, "A Randomized Trial of the Effects of Two Types of Short-Term Hypocaloric Diets on Weight Loss in Women with Polycystic Ovary Syndrome," *Fertility and Sterility* 81, no. 3 (March 2004): 630–37.

4. M. A. Cornier, "Insulin Sensitivity Determines the Effectiveness of Dietary Macronutrient Composition on Weight Loss in Obese Women," *Obesity Research* 13, no. 4 (April 2005): 703–9.

5. L. J. Moran, "Dietary Composition in Restoring Reproductive and Metabolic Physiology in Overweight Women with Polycystic Ovary Syndrome," *Journal of Clinical Endocrinology and Metabolism* 88, no. 2 (February 2003): 812–19.

6. P. G. Crosignani, "Overweight and Obese Anovulatory Patients with Polycystic Ovaries: Parallel Improvements in Anthropometric Indices, Ovarian Physiology, and Fertility Rate Induced by Diet," *Human Reproduction* 18, no. 9 (September 2003): 1928–32.

7. Barbara Rolls, *The Volumetrics Eating Plan: Techinques and Recipes for Feeling Full on Fewer Calories* (New York: Harper Paperbacks, 2007).

Chapter 4

1. National Center for Health Statistics, Centers for Disease Control, "National Health and Examination Survey," available online at www.cdc.gov/nchs/nhanes/nhanes1999-2000/nhanes99_00.htm.

2. "Report of the Dietary Guidelines Advisory Committee on Dietary Guidelines for Americans," 2005, available online at www.health.gov/dietaryguidelines/dga2005/report/default.htm.

3. www.health.harvard.edu/newsweek/Glycemic_index_ and glycemic_load_for_100_foods .htm.

4. College Medical Calculators, Cornell University Medical School, available online at www-users.med.cornell.edu/~spon/picu/calc/beecalc.htm.

5. Brian Wansink, *Mindless Eating: Why We Eat More Than We Think* (New York: Bantam, 2007).

6. American Diabetes Association, *Choose Your Foods: Exchange Lists for Diabetes*, available online at www.diabetes.org.

Chapter 5

1. American Diabetes Association, *Choose Your Foods: Exchange Lists for Diabetes*, available online at www.diabetes.org.

2. American Diabetes Association, *Food and Fitness: Carbohydrates*, available online at www .diabetes.org/food-and-fitness/food/what-can-i-eat/carbohydrates.html.

Chapter 6

1. L. J. Moran, "Ghrelin and Measures of Satiety Are Altered in Polycystic Ovary Syndrome but Not Differentially Affected by Diet Composition," *Journal of Clinical Endocrinology and Metabolism* 89, no. 7 (July 2004): 3337–44.

2. B. Pehlivavov, "Serum Leptin Levels Correlate with Clinical and Biochemical Indices of Insulin Resistance in Women with Polycystic Ovary Syndrome," *European Journal of Contraception & Reproductive Health Care* 14, no. 2 (April 2009): 153–59.

3. N. A. Georgopoulos, "Basal Metabolic Rate Is Decreased in Women with Polycystic Ovary Syndrome and Biochemical Hyperandrogenemia and Is Associated with Insulin Resistance," *Fertility and Sterility* 92, no. 1 (July 2009): 250–55.

4. T. M. Barber, "Obesity and Polycystic Ovary Syndrome," *Clinical Endocrinology* 65, no. 2 (August 2006) 137–45.

5. R. Pasquali, "Role of Changes in Dietary Habits in Polycystic Ovary Syndrome," *Reproductive Biomedicine Online* 8, no. 4 (April 2004): 431–39.

6. A. Gambineri, "Obesity and the Polycystic Ovary Syndrome," *International Journal of Obesity and Related Metabolic Disorders* 26, no. 7 (July 2002): 883–96. Thessaloniki ESHRE/ASRM–Sponsored PCOS Consensus Workshop, "Group Consensus on Infertility Treatment Related to Polycystic Ovary Syndrome," *Human Reproduction* 23 (March 2008): 462–77.

7. P. G. Crosignani, "Overweight and Obese Anovulatory Patients with Polycystic Ovaries: Parallel Improvements in Anthropometric Indices, Ovarian Physiology, and Fertility Rate Induced by Diet," *Human Reproduction* 18 (September 2003): 1928–32.

8. Check your BMI at one of the following websites: the Centers for Disease Control (www.cdc.gov/healthyweight/assessing/bmi/) and the Department of Health and Human Services of the National Institutes of Health (www.nhlbisupport.com/bmi/).

9. To calculate BMI for children and teens, use this calculator from the Centers for Disease Control: http://apps.nccd.cdc.gov/dnpabmi/.

10. R. R. Wing, "Successful Weight Loss Maintenance," *Annual Review of Nutrition* 21 (2001): 323–41. See the National Weight Control Registry at www.nwcr.ws.

11. S. Phelan, "Are the Eating and Exercise Habits of Successful Weight Losers Changing?" *Obesity* 14 (2006): 710–16.

12. R. Wing, "A Self-Regulation Program for Maintenance of Weight Loss," *New England Journal of Medicine* 355, no. 15 (October 2006): 1563–1572.

13. Anne M. Fletcher, *Thin for Life: Ten Keys to Success from People Who Have Lost Weight and Kept It Off* (Boston, MA: Houghton Mifflin Harcourt, 2003).

14. F. M. Sacks, "Comparison of Weight-Loss Diets with Different Compositions of Fat, Protein, and Carbohydrates," *New England Journal of Medicine* 360, no. 9 (February 2009): 859–73.

15. D. Paddon-Jones, "Protein, Weight Management, and Satiety," *American Journal of Clinical Nutrition* 87 (May 2008): 1558S–1561S.

16. D. K. Layman, "A Reduced Ratio of Dietary Carbohydrate to Protein Improves Body Composition and Blood Lipid Profiles during Weight Loss in Adult Women," *Journal of Nutrition* 133 (February 2003): 411–17.

17. S. E. Kasim-Karakas, "Effects of Protein versus Simple Sugar Intake on Weight Loss in Polycystic Ovary Syndrome (According to the National Institutes of Health Criteria)," *Fertility and Sterility* 92, no. 1 (July 2009): 262–70.

18. James Prochaska, *Changing for Good: A Revolutionary Six-Stage Program for Overcoming Bad Habits and Moving Your Life Positively Forward* (New York: Harper Paperbacks (September 1, 1995). W. F. Velicer, J. O. Psochaska, et al., "Detailed Overview of the Transtheoretical Model," available online at www.uri.edu/research/cprc/TTM/detailedoverview.htm.

Chapter 7

1. V. A. Hughes, "Exercise Increases Muscle GLUT-4 Levels and Insulin Action in Subjects with Impaired Glucose Tolerance," *American Journal of Physiology* 264, no. 6 (part 1) (June 1993): E855–62.

2. S. A. Dugan, "Physical Activity and Reduced Intra-Abdominal Fat in Midlife African American and White Women," *Obesity* (Silver Spring) 18, no. 6 (June 2010): 1260–5.

3. "Physical Activity and Health: A Report of the Surgeon General," available online at www .cdc.gov/NCCDPHP/SGR/summ.htm.

4. C. Vigorito, "Beneficial Effects of a Three-Month Structured Exercise Training Program on Cardiopulmonary Functional Capacity in Young Women with PCOS," *Journal of Clinical Endocrinology and Metabolism* 92, no. 4 (2007): 1379–84. F. Giallauria, "Exercise Training Improved Autonomic Function and Inflammatory Patterns in Women with PCOS," *Clinical Endocrinology* 69 (2008): 792–98.

5. F. Orio, "Metabolic and Cardiopulmonary Effect of Detraining after a Structured Exercise Training Programme in Young PCOS Women," *Clinical Endocrinology* 68 (2008): 976–81.

6. J. Tuomilehto, "Nonpharmacologic Therapy and Exercise in the Prevention of Type 2 Diabetes," *Diabetes Care* 32 supplement 2 (November 2009): S189–93.

7. "ACSM Physical Activity and Public Health Guidelines," available online at www.acsm .org/AM/Template.cfm?Section=Home_Page&TEMPLATE=/CM/HTMLDisplay .cfm&CONTENTID=7764.

8. "Physical Activity Guidelines for Americans," available online at www.health.gov/ paguidelines/.

9. D. J. Cuff, "Effective Exercise Modality to Reduce Insulin Resistance in Women with Type 2 Diabetes," *Diabetes Care* 26, no. 11 (November 2003): 2977–82.

Chapter 8

1. A. A. Ginde, "Demographic Differences and Trends of Vitamin D Insufficiency in the U.S. Population, 1988–2004," *Archives of Internal Medicine* 169, no. 6 (March 2009): 626–32.

2. M. L. Melamed, "25-hydroxyvitamin D Levels and the Risk of Mortality in the General Population," *Archives of Internal Medicine* 168, no. 15 (August 2008): 1629–37. C. H. Wilkins, "Vitamin D Deficiency Is Associated with Low Mood and Worse Cognitive Performance in Older Adults," *American Journal of Geriatric Psychiatry* 14, no. 12 (December 2006): 1032–40. M. F. Holick, "Vitamin D: A D-Lightful Health Perspective," *Nutrition Reviews* 66, no. 10 (suppl. 2) (October 2008): S182–94.

3. M. F. Holick, "The Role of Vitamin D for Bone Health and Fracture Prevention," *Current Osteoporosis Reports* 4, no. 3 (September 2006): 96–102.

4. E. Wehr, "Association of Hypovitaminosis D with Metabolic Disturbances in Polycystic Ovary Syndrome," *European Journal of Endocrinology* 161, no. 4 (October 2009): 575–82. P. Knekt, "Serum Vitamin D and Subsequent Occurrence of Type 2 Diabetes," *Epidemiology* 19, no. 5 (September 2008): 666–71.

5. P. R. Von Hurst, "Vitamin D Supplementation Reduces Insulin Resistance in South Asian Women Living in New Zealand Who Are Insulin Resistant and Vitamin D Deficient: A Randomized, Placebo-Controlled Trial," *British Journal of Nutrition* 28 (September 2009): 1–7.

6. "Osteoporosis: Peak Bone Mass in Women," available online at www.niams.nih.gov/ Health_Info/Bone/Osteoporosis/bone_mass.asp).

7. M. Van Loan, "The Role of Dairy Foods and Dietary Calcium in Weight Management," *Journal of the American College of Nutrition* 28 (suppl. 1) (February 2009): 120S–9S.

8. B. Rashidi, "The Effects of Calcium, Vitamin D, and Metformin on Polycystic Ovary Syndrome: A Pilot Study," *Taiwan Journal of Obstetrics and Gynecology* 48, no. 2 (June 2009): 142–47.

9. J. A. Greenberg, "Omega-3 Fatty Acid Supplementation during Pregnancy," *Reviews in Obstetrics and Gynecology* 1, no. 4 (Fall 2008): 162–69. J. R. Hibbelin, "Seafood Consumption, the DHA Content of Mother's Milk, and Prevalence Rates of Postpartum

Depression: A Cross-National, Ecological Analysis," *Journal of Affective Disorders* 69, nos. 1–3 (May 2002): 15–29.

10. J. Denomme, "Directly Quantifying Dietary (N-3) Fatty Acid Intakes of Pregnant Canadian Women Are Lower Than Current Dietary Recommendations," *Journal of Nutrition* 135, no. 2 (February 2005): 206–11.

11. "Omega 3 Fatty Acids during Pregnancy," March of Dimes, available online at www .marchofdimes.com/pnhec/159_55030.asp#.

12. E. L. Lien, "Toxicology and Safety of DHA," *Prostaglandins, Leukotrienes, and Essential Fatty Acids* 81, nos. 2–3 (August–September 2009): 125–32.

13. C. L. Broadhusrt, "Clinical Studies on Chromium Picolinate Supplementation in Diabetes Mellitus: A Review," *Diabetes Technology and Therapeutics* 8, no. 6 (December 2006): 677–87.

14. M. L. Lydic, "Chromium Picolinate Improves Insulin Sensitivity in Obese Subjects with Polycystic Ovary Syndrome," *Fertility and Sterility* 86, no. 1 (July 2006): 243–46.

15. N. Igbal, "Chromium Picolinate Does Not Improve Key Features of Metabolic Syndrome in Obese Nondiabetic Adults," *Metabolic Syndrome and Related Disorders* 7, no. 2 (Summer 2009): 143–50.

16. National Institutes of Health, Office of Dietary Supplements, "Dietary Supplement Fact Sheet: Chromium," available online at http://ods.od.nih.gov/factsheets/chromium.asp.

17. Natural Medicines Comprehensive Database, "Scientific Gold Standard for Evidence-Based, Clinical Information on Natural Medicines," available online at www.naturaldatabase.com.

18. J. E. Nestler, "Role of Inositolphosphoglycan Mediators of Insulin Action in the Polycystic Ovary Syndrome," *Journal of Pediatric Endocrinology and Metabolism* 13 (suppl. 5) (2000): 1295–98.

19. J. E. Nestler, "Ovulatory and Metabolic Effects of D-Chiroinositol in the Polycystic Ovary Syndrome," *New England Journal of Medicine* 340, no. 17 (April 29, 1999): 1314–20. K. I. Cheang, "Insulin-Stimulated Release of D-Chiro-Inositol-Containing Inositolphosphoglycan Mediator Correlates with Insulin Sensitivity in Women with Polycystic Ovary Syndrome," *Metabolism* 57, no. 10 (October 2008): 1390–97.

20. MIN-DAK Growers, Ltd., available online at www.minndak.com/factsofbuckwheat.htm.

21. Natural Medicines Comprehensive Database, "Scientific Gold Standard for Evidence-Based, Clinical Information on Natural Medicines," available online at www.naturaldatabase.com.

Chapter 9

1. American Heart Association, "Metabolic Syndrome," available online at www.americanheart.org/presenter.jhtml?identifier=4756.

2. American Heart Association, "What Your Cholesterol Levels Mean," available online at www.americanheart.org/presenter.jhtml?identifier=183.

3. American Heart Association, "Blood Pressure Levels," available online at www.americanheart.org/presenter.jhtml?identifier=4450.

4. American Diabetes Association, "Prediabetes FAQ," available online at www.diabetes.org/diabetes-basics/prevention/pre-diabetes/pre-diabetes-faqs.html.

5. National Heart Lung and Blood Institute, "Your Guide to Lowering Your Blood Pressure with DASH," available online at www.nhlbi.nih.gov/health/public/heart/hbp/dash/new_dash.pdf.

6. "Polycystic Ovary Syndrome: Frequently Asked Questions," womenshealth.gov, the Federal Government Source for Women's Health Information, Department of Health and Human Services, available online at www.womenshealth.gov/faq/polycystic-ovary-syndrome.cfm#j.

7. To learn more about the DASH diet and how to make it work for you, see National Heart Lung and Blood Institute's DASH website (which includes great recipes and helpful meal plans) at www.nhlbi.nih.gov/health/public/heart/hbp/dash/new_dash.pdf.

Chapter 11

1. Food Marketing Institute Supermarket Facts available online at www.fmi.org/facts_figs/?fuseaction=.

2. Food and Drug Administration, "How to Understand and Use the Nutrition Facts Label," available online at www.fda.gov/Food/LabelingNutrition/ConsumerInformation/ucm078889.htm. National Institutes of Health, "Tip Sheet for Reading Labels," available online at www.nhlbi.nih.gov/chd/Tipsheets/reading-labels-tips.htm.

3. This limit on weekly meat intake is from the American Institute for Cancer Research, "Food, Nutrition, Physical Activity, and the Prevention of Cancer: A Global Perspective—Animal Foods," available online at www.dietandcancerreport.org/?p=recommendation_05.

Chapter 12

1. Hope Warshaw, *Eat Out, Eat Right* (Berkeley, CA: Agate Surrey, 2008).

Chapter 13

1. S. C. Bishop, "Polycystic Ovary Syndrome, Depression, and Affective Disorders," *Endocrine Practice* 15, no. 5 (July–August 2009): 475–82.

2. E. Hollinrake, "Increased Risk of Depressive Disorders in Women with Polycystic Ovary Syndrome," *Fertility and Sterility* 89, no. 4 (April 2008): 1029–30.

3. H. L. Ching, "Quality of Life and Psychological Morbidity in Women with Polycystic Ovary Syndrome: Body Mass Index, Age, and the Provision of Patient Information Are Significant Modifiers," *Clinical Endocrinology* 66, no. 3 (March 2007): 373–79.

4. T. N. Akbaralt, "Dietary Pattern and Depressive Symptoms in Middle Age," *British Journal of Psychiatry* 195, no. 5 (November 2009): 408–13.

5. S. S. Lim, "Hyperandrogenemia, Psychological Distress, and Food Cravings in Young Women," *Physiology and Behavior* 98, no. 3 (September 2009): 276–80. C. L. Weiner, "Androgens and Mood Dysfunction in Women: Comparison of Women with PCOS to Healthy Controls," *Psychosomatic Medicine* 66 (2004): 356–62.

6. L. M. Liao, "Exercise and Body Image Distress in Overweight and Obese Women with Polycystic Ovary Syndrome: A Pilot Investigation," *Gynecological Endocrinology* 24, no. 10 (October 2008): 555–61.

7. http://nccam.nih.gov/health/atoz.htm.

8. http://nccam.nih.gov/health/whatiscam.

Chapter 14

1. "Dietary Guidelines for Americans 2005," available online at www.health.gov/DIETARYGUIDELINES/dga2005/document/html/chapter2.htm).

2. J. Chavarro, "Iron Intake and Risk of Ovulatory Infertility," *Obstetrics and Gynecology* 108, no. 5 (November 2006): 1145–52.

3. M. L. Mulligan, "Implications of Vitamin D Deficiency in Pregnancy and Lactation," *American Journal of Obstetrics and Gynecology* 202, no. 5 (May 2010): 429.e1–9.

4. Elizabeth Ward, conversation with author, December 12, 2009.

5. R. Pasquali, "The Impact of Obesity on Reproduction in Women with Polycystic Ovary Syndrome," *British Journal of Obstetrics and Gynecology: An International Journal of Obstetrics and Gynecology* 113, no. 10 (October 2006): 1148–59.

6. "Folic Acid," March of Dimes, available online at www.marchofdimes.com/pnhec/173_769 .asp.

7. "Omega-3 Fatty Acids during Pregnancy," March of Dimes, available online at www.marchofdimes.com/pnhec/159_55030.asp.

8. F. H. Nawaz and others, "Does Continuous Use of Metformin throughout Pregnancy Improve Pregnancy Outcomes in Women with Polycystic Ovarian Syndrome?" *Journal of Obstetrics and Gynaecology Research* 34, no. 5 (October 2008): 832–37.

9. "Caffeine and Pregnancy," March of Dimes, available online at www.marchofdimes.com/ professionals/14332_1148.asp.

10. H. Klonoff-Cohen, "A Prospective Study of the Effects of Female and Male Caffeine Consumption on the Reproductive Endpoints of IVF and Gamete Intra-Fallopian Transfer," *Human Reproduction* 17, no. 7 (July 2002): 1746–54.

11. "Diabetes in Pregnancy," March of Dimes, available online at www.marchofdimes.com/ professionals/19695_1197.asp.

12. American Dietetic Association, "Position Paper: Nutrition and Lifestyle for a Healthy Pregnancy Outcome," *Journal of the American Dietetic Association* 208 (2008): 553–61.

13. Institute of Medicine, "Weight Gain during Pregnancy: Reexamining the Guidelines," available online at www.iom.edu/-/media/Files/Report%20Files/2009/Weight-Gain-During-Pregnancy-Reexamining-the-Guidelines/Report%20Brief%20-%20Weight%20 Gain%20During%20Pregnancy.ashx.

Index